THE LIVING WILL

Joseph E. Beltran
D. Min.

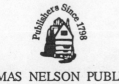

Publishers Since 1798

THOMAS NELSON PUBLISHERS
Nashville

Published in Nashville, Tennessee, by Thomas Nelson Publishers, Inc.

Scripture quotations are from the NEW REVISED STANDARD VERSION of the Bible, © 1989, by the Division of Christian Education of the National Council of the Churches of Christ in the United States of America.

"The Medical Directive" (1) © 1990 by Linda L. Emanuel and Ezekiel J. Emanuel. The authors of this form advise that it should be completed pursuant to a discussion between the principal and his or her physician, so that the principal can be adequately informed of any pertinent medical information, and so that the physician can be apprised of the intentions of the principal and the existence of such a document which may be made part of the principal's medical records. (2) This form was originally published as part of an article by Linda L. Emanuel and Ezekiel J. Emanuel, "The Medical Directive: A New Comprehensive Advance Care Document" in *Journal of the American Medical Association*, June 9, 1989;261:3290. It does not reflect the official policy of the American Medical Association. Used by permission.

This publication is designed to provide accurate and authoritative information in regard to the subject matter covered. It is sold with the understanding that the publisher is not engaged in rendering legal, accounting, or other professional service. If legal advice or other expert assistance is required, the services of a competent professional should be sought.

From a Declaration of Principles jointly adopted by a Committee of the American Bar Association and a Committee of Publishers and Associations.

Library of Congress Cataloging-in-Publication Data

Beltran, Joseph E.

The living will and other life-and-death medical choices / Joseph E. Beltran.

   p. cm.

Includes bibliographical references.

ISBN 0-8407-6746-3

   1. Right to die. 2. Right to die—Law and legislation. 3. Right to die—Religious aspects. I. Title.

R726.8.B44 1993

362.1'75—dc20   93-27177
                                                     CIP

Published in the United States of America

1 2 3 4 5 6 7 — 99 98 97 96 95 94

To my wife, Kathy,
who is my mentor,
best friend,
and traveling companion.
You are the love of my life.

CONTENTS

ACKNOWLEDGMENTS

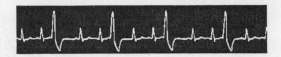

It would not have been possible to write this book without having had the experience of living through extremely difficult decisions with so many families whose loved ones live at Fairview Developmental Center. Their commitment to make the best possible decisions for their family members continues to give me new insights into the way decisions concerning life-sustaining treatment should be made.

I also gratefully acknowledge the following people:

The members of the bioethics committee at Fairview Developmental Center and those colleagues on the steering committee of the Orange County Bioethics Network whose wisdom and insight have greatly enhanced this book.

Donald Brandenburgh, whose integrity and tireless perseverance as a literary agent make him an author's greatest ally.

Amanda and Stephen Sorenson, whose skillful editing has helped convey this important information about life-sustaining medical treatment and advance directives.

Ronald N. Haynes, who supported this project from the beginning and whose efforts ensured that the message of this book would be told.

PREFACE

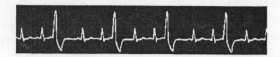

You're involved in a serious car accident. Paramedics arrive on the scene after you have been without oxygen for ten minutes. You are resuscitated but never regain consciousness. Two neurologists diagnose you as being in a persistent vegetative state, meaning you'll never regain an awareness of your surroundings. Because you cannot swallow, the only way doctors can keep you alive is to place a feeding tube directly into your stomach.

Thought: *If you were in this situation, would you want to be kept alive with the feeding tube?*

Or, suddenly and unexpectedly, you begin to feel dizzy and get a severe headache at work one day. A friend rushes you to the hospital. The emergency room doctors determine you have had a brain-damaging stroke. While in the emergency room, you lose consciousness. The physicians then determine that you are in a coma and have only a slight chance of recovery.

Thought: *Would you want to be kept alive in this comatose condition through artificial nutrition and hydration? Or would you want all treatment stopped, except those procedures that make you comfortable?*

What if you should learn that you have acute leukemia? Your physician tells you that recent technology has improved the likelihood of a long-term cure, but the treatment procedure is long and painful. It includes chemotherapy, which means three weeks in the hospital, probable infection, and hair loss. More chemotherapy will also be needed a few weeks later. If you make it through the course of treatment with good results, you'll need a complicated, often painful, bone-marrow transplant. Combined, these procedures have a 25 percent chance of success for a complete cure. Without treatment, you'll probably die within a matter of weeks.

Thought: What would you do in this situation? What factors would influence your decision? Why?

Maybe you are eighty years old and live in a skilled nursing facility. You are no longer ambulatory and must use a wheelchair. One day you develop a serious infection that can be easily treated and are transferred to an acute care hospital. When you are admitted, a nurse asks you what your preference is regarding cardiopulmonary resuscitation (CPR) in the event your heart or lungs stop working while you are hospitalized.

Thought: Would you ask that a Do Not Resuscitate order (no CPR) be written in your medical record? Why or why not?

These hypothetical scenarios are just a few of the actual clinical situations that arise every day. These illustrations point out the need for each of us to think about life-sustaining issues and to discuss them with family members, friends, and the people who will be our surrogates for health care decisions.

Increasing advances in sophisticated medical technology enable doctors to keep almost anyone "alive"—respirating and circulating—indefinitely. Of course, being "alive" is the prerequisite for all human rights. Most of us would agree that the protection of our human rights is of enormous importance. "Saving" or "prolonging" or "sustaining" life is commonly viewed as a way of protecting our rights as human beings. I believe this is a simplistic interpretation of a complex ethical issue. Is saving, prolonging, or sustaining life *always* the right action to take in the interest of protecting human rights? When, if ever, is it appropriate to say, "Halt. Enough is enough."? When does a patient, or a patient's family, have the right to say that what *can* be done *need not* be done, or perhaps even *ought not* to be done?

Fifteen years elapsed between the time of Karen Ann Quinlan's tragic mishap in 1975, the car accident that permanently disabled Nancy Cruzan in 1983, and the court's resolution of the Cruzan case in 1990. During that time a societal consensus evolved concerning the right of a patient or a patient's family to refuse or to stop life-sustaining medical treatment. On December 1, 1991, this consensus became the law of the land. Named The Patient Self-Determination Act, this federal legislation requires health care providers to inform all patients in writing of their right to refuse unwanted medical treatment and their right to formulate a document called an advance directive.

These changes in our approach to medical decision making call each of us to consider the risks related to these issues. Beyond that, these changes urge us to make and document our desires and decisions concerning life-sustaining medical treatment. The primary objective of this book is to create an awareness of medical treatment issues and to show you how you can respond appropriately. This book strives to be ecumenical in spirit, drawing on both Christian faith traditions as they relate to medical treatment decisions and on an emerging body of related secular literature.

I wrote this book with five goals in mind:

First, to give you a basic and understandable overview of bioethics. Together, we'll consider where our society has come from, where it is now, and where the future might lead us in regard to life-sustaining treatment and related decisions concerning individual freedom, self-determination, and health care. In order to gain historical perspective, we will first examine both the Quinlan and Cruzan cases, which established important ethical and legal precedents. We will then explore the ethical, legal and theological issues and concerns surrounding decisions to withhold or withdraw life-sustaining treatment. We will also consider the role of spirituality in illness, dying, and death.

Second, to consider our individual rights to refuse unwanted medical treatment and to explore ways to exercise those rights. We'll learn what an advance directive is and analyze the features of each of the three types of advance directives. Because exploring personal values in relation to medical treatment is part of writing an advance directive, we'll see how to evaluate and document those values. Samples of the types of advance directives discussed, as well as a values history inventory and a medical directive that can be used to consider personal treatment preferences, are included. Finally, we'll be able to write the type of directive that best suits our needs.

Third, to enable individuals to make sound ethical decisions regarding withholding or withdrawing life-sustaining medical treatment. We'll also explore how those decisions can be grounded in Christian principles and in the emerging societal consensus.

Fourth, to challenge all of us to exercise greater control over our medical care to ensure that our wishes will be known and followed if we become unable to make competent medical treatment decisions. I've tried to make this information easy to understand so that readers will be better able to make informed decisions concerning medical treatment.

Fifth, to provide resources that will help us—and those we love—face serious illness and death.

Finally, I'd like to share my credentials and motivation for writing this book. I am an ordained minister in the Presbyterian Church (USA) and began working as a Protestant chaplain for the State of California at Fairview Developmental Center in May, 1985. As one of seven residential centers operated by the Department of Developmental Services of the State of California, Fairview provides services to individuals who have developmental disabilities and who require our structured living environment. Fairview currently provides services to approximately 1,100 developmentally disabled people who also have some form of mental retardation. Most of them are severely or profoundly disabled and have multiple handicapping conditions.

I became a member of the bioethics committee at Fairview in 1985 and began examining the issue of withdrawing life-sustaining support as it related to our vulnerable patient population. In 1987, I was appointed chairperson of the committee, which has since provided case consultation for more than one hundred patients in circumstances which made us consider foregoing some forms of medical treatment. Since 1987 I have also been a member of the steering committee of the Orange County Bioethics Network, which encourages communication between various bioethics committees and conducts education programs on topics of current interest.

One of my responsibilities as chaplain at Fairview is to assist family members with funeral arrangements when necessary. This gives me a unique perspective on medical ethics. Most ethicists are moral philosophers or physicians. My vantage point is different because I am an ethicist who participates in aspects of patients' cases from the outset through the funeral. I have also done advanced study in bioethics to supplement my hands-on experience with patients and families. My doctoral project dealt specifically with the ethics of foregoing medical treatment of mentally retarded persons.

It is important to note that I do not direct this volume solely, or even primarily, to senior citizens. Although death may seem more imminent to senior citizens, the decision to write an advance directive—and what to include in it—is pertinent to all of us. Accidents and illnesses come as thieves in the night and do not choose their victims on the basis of age, race, gender, or any other variable.

CHAPTER 1

Two Women
Who Challenged
Our Thinking

The names and stories of two young women, Karen Ann Quinlan and Nancy Beth Cruzan, have been burned into the collective memory of America. Vibrant young women in their prime, their lives were changed forever by tragic circumstances which permanently altered their lives and the lives of their families and friends. *Quinlan* and *Cruzan* have thus come to represent our struggles, as individuals and as a society, with ultimate medical and ethical questions concerning the "gray areas" of our lives.

Medical technology is growing at a tremendous rate and at great financial cost to all of us. It has also exacted a high cost in human suffering. Powerful technologies are capable of sustaining basic biological life—respiration and circulation—almost indefinitely, yet such life may be void of any possibility for self-awareness or social interaction.

Many complex questions and ethical dilemmas accompany our technology's ability to prolong life. Although advancing medical technology has enabled us to prolong life far beyond what we ever imagined, there is a limit to what medicine can accomplish. For example, life expectancy lengthens every year as medical technology improves. But with the capabilities of modern medicine to provide a "quantity" of life come challenges and questions about the quality of such life. Each time a new treatment is developed and routinely practiced, perplexing ethical questions also arise.

> Doctors call it the Daedalus effect, after the Greek architect who was imprisoned in the labyrinth, the maze he himself designed. It was the fate of Daedalus, as it is perhaps the fate of doctors and scientists and anyone pursuing progress, that every time he solves a problem, a new one was created.[1]

As citizens and as a society, we should ask ourselves what we are accomplishing by the apparent quest to ultimately defeat death through technological advances. We should ask whether the goal is worth the emotional and financial cost. We need to determine when enough is enough.

In order to address these questions, each of us must explore our personal value systems in relation to the sophisticated medical treatment available. New medical technologies compel us to ask ourselves:

- "What are we truly doing when we intervene to stave off death?"
- "Which values are we seeking to serve?"
- "How do we formulate those values?"
- "Which basic principles define our well-being as a community?"
- "Should we sustain life when the recipient arguably gains little or nothing?"
- "Would we want our own lives sustained by machines and feeding tubes?"

- "What limitations on medical treatment do we desire?"
- "What is the best way to document our wishes before we become seriously ill?"

The cases of Karen Ann Quinlan and Nancy Beth Cruzan serve as examples of some of the treatment questions we face. These two women represent hundreds of litigations and literally thousands of patients for whom treatment/non-treatment decisions are made each year. Let's consider each case separately.

Karen Ann Quinlan

In April, 1975, twenty-one-year-old Karen Ann Quinlan returned home from a party and went to bed not feeling well. During the night she lapsed into a coma-like state and never awoke. An electroencephalogram revealed that half of her brain had totally stopped functioning due to massive brain damage; the other half gave off slight but steady signals.

During the next few months, Karen Ann lost sixty pounds and slowly curled into a fetal position. A ventilator assisted her breathing and an intravenous tube supplied her food. Her prognosis was grim: her chance of regaining consciousness was almost nonexistent and, if she did, she would be severely disabled mentally and physically. The ventilator seemed to prolong her inevitable death and kept her in a vegetative "twilight zone."

When her parents Joseph and Julia Quinlan, in consultation with their parish priest, requested that the hospital wean Karen Ann from the ventilator, she became the focus of an international media frenzy. Photographs of Karen Ann and her parents, as well as cryptic accounts of her case, appeared

3

in the media worldwide. Talk show hosts probed the intricacies of such concepts as "ordinary" versus "extraordinary" means of life-sustaining treatment and the rights of all individuals to life, privacy, and self-determination. The November 3, 1975 cover of *Newsweek* boldly asked, "A Right to Die?"

The Quinlans wanted their daughter to either breathe on her own, which was highly unlikely, or to be allowed to die peacefully. The hospital steadfastly refused the family's request. Hospital officials were concerned that removing the ventilator might constitute immoral and illegal "mercy killing"—the direct and intentional suffocation of a severely handicapped and defenseless person.

After the hospital denied their request, the Quinlans took the case to a lower New Jersey court, which upheld the hospital's interpretation that prolonging Karen Ann's life was in the best interest of all concerned. On March 31, 1976, almost a year after her accident, the New Jersey Supreme Court overruled the lower court and decided in favor of the Quinlan family.

Basing its decision on the "right to privacy," the New Jersey Supreme Court ruled that the hospital had overstepped its bounds by invading the privacy of Karen Ann or, in her present unconscious state, the privacy of the Quinlans as guardians and surrogates. The Court also stated that persons who carry out familial instructions are legally immune from criminal prosecution. Although a number of ethicists and jurists disagreed with the "privacy" defense, considering it too broad and open to potential patient abuse, most agreed that the decision to remove Karen Ann from the ventilator was indeed justified.

Respectful of the ethical code and integrity of the hospital that had refused to remove the ventilator, the Quinlan family had Karen Ann transferred to another health care facility, which acquiesced to the family's wishes and weaned her from ventilator dependence. Ironically, Karen Ann continued to breathe independently. Her brain stem was apparently healthy enough to sustain her basic respiratory and circulatory functions. Unwilling to press the case to have artificially administered fluids and nutrition removed, Karen Ann's parents faithfully attended her for the next ten years. They arranged for her to receive care in a long-term, skilled nursing facility and visited her regularly. Although they had been willing to allow her to die if she could not breathe on her own, they were determined to care for her in her ongoing condition.

On June 11, 1985, more than ten years after the initial incident, Karen Ann died, never having regained consciousness. The toll in personal pain for Karen Ann seemed nonexistent, but the physical, mental, and emotional anguish of her family and professional care givers was tremendous. The ethical questions call us to consider whether she was unfairly kept from dying during the decade of artificially administered nutrition and hydration. Was it "right" to sustain her life in that way? Should she have been allowed a peaceful, dignified death?

Nancy Beth Cruzan

At 12:54 a.m. on January 11, 1983, a Missouri state trooper was dispatched to the scene of a single-car accident in rural Jasper County. Arriving six minutes later, Officer Dale Penn found twenty-five-year-old Nancy Beth Cruzan lying face down in a ditch. She had been thrown approximately thirty-five feet from her car. When Officer Penn checked her vital signs, she had lost cardiac and respiratory function. At 1:09 a.m., paramedics arrived and restored her cardiac function and spontaneous respiration within three minutes. The best estimate of her period of cardiac arrest and oxygen deprivation was a minimum of twelve to fourteen minutes. She was then admitted into an acute-care hospital. In order to ease the feeding process, doctors surgically implanted a gastrostomy tube directly into her stomach to provide nutrition and hydration.

Nancy was later transferred to a long-term care facility operated by the State of Missouri. She was diagnosed as being in a persistent vegetative state. She was not brain dead but was severely brain damaged. Although her eyes were often open, she remained "oblivious to her environment except for reflexive responses to sound and perhaps pain stimuli."[2] Only her brain stem (the lower portion of the brain which controls the autonomic functions of breathing and circulation) was functioning. Her thinking mind was permanently obliterated and her body locked in a fetal position. Medical personnel estimated her life expectancy to be approximately thirty years, if they treated her condition aggressively.

Over the course of the next few years, valiant efforts to rehabilitate her proved fruitless. Her respiration and circulation were not artificially maintained, but she had little or no cognitive or reflexive ability to swallow food or water and there was no prognosis that she would ever regain those functions. Her total nutritional intake—a predigested, fortified liquid diet—was administered through the gastrostomy tube.

After five years of coping with Nancy's medical, psychological, moral, and legal "limbo"—suspended somewhere between the living and the dead—her parents, Joe and Joyce Cruzan, petitioned a Missouri trial court to discontinue artificial feeding. They wanted to remove the feeding tube in order to allow Nancy to finish the dying process that began in 1983 when her heart stopped and her brain was deprived of oxygen. Missouri Probate Judge Charles Teel granted an order to remove the feeding tube. But, Missouri's attorney general appealed the decision to the State Supreme Court. The higher court reversed Teel's ruling and determined that the state's interest in preserving life demanded "clear and convincing evidence" that an incompetent patient, such as Nancy Cruzan, would have chosen to terminate treatment. In other words, distinct and verifiable proof of Nancy's prior desires and preferences was necessary in order for the State of Missouri to relinquish its presumed interest in preserving life. The case was then appealed to the United States Supreme Court. In a 5-4 decision, issued on June 25, 1990, the Supreme Court affirmed the "principle that a competent person has a constitutionally protected liberty interest in refusing unwanted medical treatment."[3] Nonetheless, the majority opinion determined that our United States Constitution does not forbid states from requiring "clear and convincing evidence" of an incompetent patient's prior wishes regarding the withdrawal of life-sustaining treatment. The Court further determined that evidence submitted to Judge Teel could be deemed insufficient to fulfill the State of Missouri's requirement for being "clear and convincing."

Thus the U.S. Supreme Court upheld the Missouri Supreme Court's decision to refuse the Cruzan family's request, based on the premise that there was insufficient evidence of Nancy's prior wishes. All of this took place without denying a competent patient the right to refuse treatment; without denying that some states may have fewer stringent restrictions on determining noncompetent patients' prior wishes; and without denying that some states may choose to apply a generic "best interest" or "reasonable person" standard rather than attempt to prove a patient's prior wishes.

Subsequently, the Cruzans provided further evidence of Nancy's prior values and wishes to Judge Teel, who deemed the evidence "clear and convincing" and granted the Cruzans' renewed petition. Missouri's attorney general did not contest this second decision by Judge Teel and the feeding tube was withdrawn. On December 26, 1990, almost seven years after her car accident, Nancy died. She remained in a persistent vegetative state until her death, although she did exhibit intermittent grimacing if jabbed, poked, or given painful stimuli. The grief of her family, their tensions with state health care employees, and the tensions among the employees have been well-documented, but the ethical questions remain. Was it unfair to deny Nancy Cruzan a peaceful death? Was it "right" to prolong her life?

CHAPTER 2

Making Medical Treatment Decisions

A medical, legal, religious, and ethical consensus regarding medical treatment has been emerging in the United States since 1976. This consensus has been confirmed by the U.S. Supreme Court in the Cruzan decision and by the U.S. Congress in the 1990 passage of the Patient Self-Determination Act. In its most basic form, the consensus is this: *A competent patient can refuse any proposed medical treatment at any time if he or she deems it not to be in his or her best interest.* The patient's personal judgment should be respected in determining whether a given treatment is worthwhile to the patient in a given situation.

State courts have repeatedly affirmed the right of competent adults to determine for themselves the kind of health care they wish to receive or refuse. The following excerpt from a court decision in 1914 clearly expresses the legal consensus:

Every human being of adult years and sound mind has a right to determine what shall be done with his own body; and a surgeon who performs an operation without his patient's consent commits an assault, for which he is liable in damages.[1]

This principle is generally referred to as the right to *informed consent*. Informed consent gives us the right to oversee our own physical and mental well-being and to grant permission before a physician, therapist, dentist, pharmacist, or other health care professional can proceed with any treatment. Most of us have given consent for some type of medical procedure, whether it was having a tooth filled, taking a prescription drug, or undergoing a surgical procedure.

The right to refuse medical treatment is the converse side of the reasonable exercise of informed consent. If we do not want a particular treatment, it ought not be forced on us against our wishes, provided we are legally competent to make such a judgment. Any competent patient who has the ability to understand his or her medical condition and to make informed choices has the right to refuse any medical treatment. This right to consent to or to refuse medical treatment continues even when we are no longer able to make decisions for ourselves. The rights to life and self-determination are inherent and abiding. Patients who lack decision-making capacity have the same fundamental right to determine the course of their medical treatment as patients who have decision-making capacity.

The concept of self-determination is one of the foundational principles in the emerging consensus on medical treatment decisions. A second aspect of the consensus focuses around the issue of what constitutes ethical medical treatment. The principle of proportionality, meaning whether the benefits of a treatment justify the burden of that treatment to the patient, is the primary means used to decide whether a specific treatment should be administered. Let's briefly consider the major elements of the emerging medical, legal, religious, and ethical consensus concerning decisions about life-sustaining treatment.

Any Patient Has the Right to Consent to or to Refuse Any Medical Treatment at Any Time

Treatment decisions should be an expression of an individual's personal choice and should be made after analyzing medical information provided by health care professionals. Decisions to withhold or withdraw life-sustaining treatment are essentially value decisions, and different people will use different value systems to reach their decisions. Therefore, the controlling factor in making decisions regarding medical care should be the patient's unique system of values and preferences.

Patients May Exercise Their Right to Self-Determination Through Surrogate Decision Makers

Patients who lose the capacity to make informed decisions have the same fundamental right to determine the course of their medical treatment as do competent patients. When a once-competent patient becomes noncompetent, the right to self-determination passes to a surrogate decision maker if one is available. If a noncompetent patient's desires regarding medical treatment are known, they should be followed.

Patients may express their treatment desires through an advance directive document, which may name a surrogate who is empowered to make treatment decisions for the patient. If patients do not express their treatment desires while competent, or if they never were capable of making informed decisions, then it is still appropriate for surrogate decision makers to make treatment decisions on behalf of noncompetent patients.

A surrogate should be someone who knows the patient well, such as a family member, a significant other, or a close friend. A surrogate may be:

1. a named proxy
2. a conservator who has specific powers to make medical decisions
3. a family member
4. a close friend.

The surrogate's decisions should be guided by: a patient's Living Will, Durable Power of Attorney for Health Care, or similar document, if one exists; other evidence of the patient's previously expressed values or treatment desires; and the best interest of the patient, which is the standard the courts have used as determined by the burdens and benefits of any treatment given to the patient.

All Medical Treatments Are to Be Analyzed According to the Principle of Proportionality

The consensus clearly rests on a crucial ethical principle: proportionality. This principle means that the burdens and benefits of any proposed treatment are evaluated, and only treatment that provides a net gain for the patient is considered to be ethical. This principle can be evaluated for an individual patient by asking the question, "Do the expected outcomes justify the burdens the patient will be expected to endure?"

In the early days of bioethics, some people believed there was a difference between not giving medical treatment and stopping a treatment that had already been started. Today, most ethicists believe there is no difference between these actions. To withhold (not start) treatment and to withdraw (take away an existing treatment or an aspect of existing treatment, such as a feeding tube) are ethically equivalent. However, all medical treatment has to be justified. If a treatment is not providing some benefit—some overall net gain—for the patient, it is not ethically justifiable.

The current legal opinion and secular consensus is that all medical treatments are to be considered equally. This means that artificial feeding is to be viewed on a level with any other medical treatment, such as cardiopulmonary resuscitation (CPR), assisted ventilation, dialysis, and antibiotic therapy. Within the religious community, however, some people would say that provision of nutrition and hydration is a basic requirement of human life and, therefore, should not be considered a medical treatment.

Of course, people disagree on what provides benefit or net gain for a patient. Some people, for instance, demand treatment that physicians believe is medically futile, that will not lead to greater benefits for the patient. In other cases, a very painful treatment could be justified if it would almost certainly lead to the patient's full cure. Despite differences of opinion on how much benefit a patient may gain from a given treatment, the principle of proportionality is valid.

Decisions in which there is no clear surrogate, or decisions regarding the withdrawal of artificial nutrition and hydration, should be made with the advisory assistance of an institutional ethics committee, which can provide a forum

> in which difficult cases can be discussed without the expense and lengthy process of a full judicial review.

There is an ethical distinction between deliberately killing a patient and letting a seriously ill patient die. Therefore, the intention of every treatment decision must be scrutinized to assure that the decision is ethically justifiable. Allowing an underlying medical condition to take a person's life is not deliberate killing and is justifiable. It is never justifiable to deliberately kill a person. For example, if a person is suffering great pain from terminal cancer, it is appropriate for a health care professional to give sufficient pain medication to alleviate the suffering, even if such a dosage may bring death more quickly. If in the same circumstances medication is given with the intent to kill, however, the act is morally wrong even if the motive is compassion.

The challenge that lies before us as individuals and as a society is the implementation of this consensus in clinical practice. The U.S. Supreme Court ruling in the Cruzan case addresses the process whereby we guarantee, enforce, and protect our right to self-determination regarding medical treatment. The Court reaffirmed our right to make our own health care decisions. It also established our right to make a written declaration regarding medical treatment in advance of a time when we may no longer have decision-making capacity. Furthermore, the court gave individual states the ability to require patients to provide "clear and convincing evidence" of their values concerning medical treatment.

The Patient Self-Determination Act

The Patient Self-Determination Act of 1990 (PSDA) was enacted to encourage people to consider their personal values and to take responsibility for their medical treatment through advance directives for medical care in the event they become noncompetent. The PSDA upholds and respects state laws concerning the use of advance directives for medical care. In many ways, the PSDA formalizes the societal consensus. The legislation seeks to take decisions concerning life-sustaining treatment out of the courts and place them within the context of each patient's personal values.

The PSDA of 1990 modifies the federal law known as the Social Security Act, specifically the provisions pertaining to the Medicare program. Effective December 1, 1991, the PSDA of 1990 requires any health care organization that is a Medicare provider—acute hospital, skilled nursing facility, home health agency, hospice program, prepaid health organization—to ensure patients' rights to participate in and direct in the health care decisions affecting themselves. Virtually every doctor, HMO, and the like in the United States receives reimbursement from Medicare, which is why this program was chosen as the vehicle by which to inform patients of their rights.

The PSDA of 1990 uses the vehicle of the advance directive as a tool to expand communication between patients and health care professionals. An advance directive is defined as a written instruction, such as a Living Will or Durable Power of Attorney for Health Care, that is recognized by the courts of the state in which the patient is being treated and that relates to the provision of care when the individual who wrote the instruction becomes incapacitated.[2] All patients receiving services from a Medicare provider must be informed in writing of their right to accept or refuse medical or surgical treatment and their right to formulate an advance directive.

Specifics of Public Law 101-508

Medicare providers are required to do the following:

1. Maintain written policies and procedures which ensure that written information is provided to patients regarding the following:
   a. Their rights as recognized by the courts of the state where they are being treated to make decisions regarding medical care, including the right to accept or to refuse medical or surgical treatment and the right to formulate advance directives; and
   b. Provider's maintenance of written policy and procedure that ensures respect for a patient's right to accept or to refuse medical treatment;
2. Document in each patient's medical record whether the individual has written an advance directive;
3. Refrain from determining levels of care or otherwise discriminating against an individual based on whether he or she has written an advance directive;
4. Ensure compliance with state law (both statutory and relevant case law) respecting advance directives; and
5. Provide staff members and the community with education on issues concerning advance directives.

The PSDA of 1990 also states that patients are to be informed of their rights under this law by virtually any health care organization. In the same way in which persons being arrested by the police must have the Miranda Rights read to them (the right to remain silent, the right to legal representation, etc.), patients now must be informed of their right to fully participate in decisions concerning life-sustaining medical treatment and their right to document their values in an advance directive. The PSDA of 1990 specifies the following guidelines for informing patients of their rights:

1. Acute hospitals must inform patients at the time of their inpatient admission.
2. Skilled nursing facilities must inform patients at the time of their admission as residents.
3. Each home health agency must inform patients when they are taken "under the care" of the agency.
4. Hospice programs must inform patients at the time they initially receive hospice care.
5. Prepaid health organizations must inform patients at the time of their enrollment.

The intention and the spirit of the PSDA of 1990 is to move the physician/patient relationship in the direction of a shared partnership by encouraging communication between physicians and patients and by encouraging patients to document their values concerning life-sustaining medical treatment. Physicians have an obligation to provide accurate clinical information. Such data includes, but is not limited to, accurate diagnosis and prognosis, the treatment options available, and the expected outcomes of various treatments. Patients are to make informed decisions concerning their own treatment based on their unique personal values and priorities. Such a partnership can empower patients and surrogates to make difficult decisions regarding life-sustaining treatment. This is in keeping with the emerging consensus on medical treatment decisions, which clearly advocates a partnership between health care professionals and patients. Decisions regarding medical treatments, particularly the decision to refuse or to withdraw life-sustaining support, require a strong collaboration between health care professionals and the decision makers.

An advance directive is the vehicle by which patients can communicate their treatment wishes. It assures that patients' constitutionally protected, abiding right to refuse or accept medical treatment is respected. It can help physicians better understand their patients' values and can help patients clarify those values. It can encourage the mutual trust and respect necessary for health care professionals and patients to make health care decisions today.

It is my opinion that every adult should execute an advance directive. The information presented in this book provides a basic overview of the issues involved in making treatment decisions, particularly as they relate to decisions to forego life-sustaining treatment. If we each take the time to become familiar with these issues and write an advanced directive, we will take much of the controversy and heartache out of gut-wrenching treatment choices, should they become necessary.

CHAPTER 3

Ethical and Theological Foundations

When the Supreme Court Justices ruled in the Cruzan case in 1990, and the U.S. Congress passed the Patient Self-Determination Act in 1990, they reflected a consensus that has been developing for many years. By studying the foundations of the current consensus, we can discover how decisions to limit life-sustaining treatment are made. We can explore the bioethical issues and the decision- making process involved for adults who have the ability to make informed decisions and once-competent but now noncompetent adults who have written advance directives.

In 1969, the Institute of Society, Ethics, and the Life Sciences (better known as The Hastings Center) was established in Hastings-On-Hudson, New York. Since its inception, The Hastings Center has functioned as an influential educational organization on the cutting edge of ethical issues. In 1973, the first edition of the *Hastings Center Report* pointed out the problems and dilemmas of medical technology:

> Remarkable advances are being made in organ transplantation, human experimentation, prenatal diagnosis of

genetic disease, the prolongation of life and control of human behavior—and each advance has posed difficult problems requiring that scientific knowledge be matched by ethical insight.[1]

In 1987, The Hastings Center published Guidelines on the Termination of Life-Sustaining Treatment and the Care of the Dying. This report was developed after extensive study of current medical and legal trends, case law, and consultation with ethicists and social scientists. In a clear and concise format, the report represents the secular component of the emerging medical, legal, and ethical consensus concerning the limitation of life-sustaining treatment. Its guidelines reflect the findings of similar studies such as the *President's Commission for the Study of Ethical Problems in Medicine and Biomedical and Behavioral Research* and those reported in numerous medical journals.

Because different sectors of the religious community have taken an interest in life-sustaining issues, there is a religious component of the consensus as well. The Roman Catholic Church, for instance, has studied these issues longer and in more detail than any group within the Christian and secular communities. Even though religious discussions concerning life-sustaining treatment are generated by different faith groups and denominations, they generally echo the secular voices. For the most part, the religious and secular conclusions are more similar than different.

When the secular and religious bodies of literature on bioethics are evaluated together, certain principles emerge that show a consistent and systematic process to be followed in order to resolve bioethical dilemmas. When decision making follows this process, patient self-determination is protected and the integrity of health care professionals is respected.

The Hastings Center's *Guidelines on the Termination of Life-Sustaining Treatment and the Care of the Dying* recognizes the complexities and nuances involved in decisions relating to the limitation of life-sustaining treatment. The report recognizes that medical, legal, and ethical decisions must be made in such cases:

> These decisions also have an inevitable social dimension. The specific decisions and the decision-making process have social, economic, and moral consequences that affect our society as a whole. They compel us, as a society, to examine our ethical priorities—our respect for life, our respect for individual autonomy and dignity, and our understanding of the ultimate goals of medicine. They confront us with issues of justice, equity, and the economic constraints on the use of scarce medical resources.[2]

More than anything else, decisions to limit life-sustaining treatment force us to define what we consider to be the ultimate goal of medicine: to provide healing and, when healing is no longer possible, to provide a caring presence. Accomplishing this goal requires a commitment to continued involvement with and support of patients when life-sustaining treatment can no longer provide any positive benefit to the patients.

Self-Determination and Competent Adults

To refuse medical treatment or to withdraw or withhold life-sustaining procedures is a basic and fundamental right of any adult who has the ability to understand his or her medical diagnosis, condition, and prognosis. Therefore, decisions that affect one's body are the most personal of all decisions. Each of us will approach such decisions from a slightly different perspective, depending on our unique set of personal values.

> No set of guidelines can or should eliminate the need to respect each patient's unique values and needs; treatment decisions must be made on a case-by-case basis after carefully assessing the benefits and burdens the health care options entail.[3]

In keeping with this viewpoint, the President's Commission for the Study of Ethical Problems in Medicine and Biomedical and Behavioral Research published a landmark report in 1983, entitled *Deciding to Forego Life-Sustaining Treatment: Ethical, Medical, and Legal Issues in Treatment Decisions*. After years of careful study, the Commission formulated the best thinking of the time and set a standard for institutional ethics committees and institutional policy. The Commission concluded that the voluntary choice of a competent and informed patient should determine the course of treatment:

> The Commission argued that decisions about the treatments that best promote a patient's health and well-being must be based on the particular patient's values and goals; no uniform, objective determination can be adequate— whether defined by society or by health care professionals.
> Respect for the self-determination of competent patients is of special importance in decisions to forego life-sustaining treatment because different people will have markedly different needs and concerns during the final period of their lives.[4]

Health care professionals serve patients best by maintaining a perspective in favor of sustaining life while recognizing that competent patients are entitled to choose to forego any treatments, including those that sustain life. Treatment decisions are patient-value decisions, made on the basis of medical data provided by health care professionals.

Wisdom can be seen in the Commission's broad conclusions. Consider, for example, the diversity that exists among the present population of the United States. Different cultures and religions view the meaning of illness and death in a variety of ways. With the great variety of cultural and religious influences present in our country, we can easily see that no blanket governmental regulation will suffice. In order to protect the principles upon which this country was founded, decisions regarding life-sustaining treatment must necessarily respect the diverse beliefs and desires of individuals. The freedoms of personal expression protected by the U.S. Constitution logically affect medical decisions as well.

The Roman Catholic Church, with its long and rich tradition of considering the moral and theological implications of medical treatment, also supports the principle of self-determination. In 1980, the Vatican restated the tradition in its "Declaration on Euthanasia," prepared by the Sacred Congregation for the Doctrine of the Faith, May 5, 1980. This document briefly summarizes the Roman Catholic Church's teaching on medical treatment from the time of Aquinas to the present. Simply stated, the consensus of this teaching is that each person is responsible to nurture life, which is a gift from God. Therefore, all people are to consider their lives as being bound closely to the will of God, the Giver of all life, not as something to be disposed of at will.

> Everyone has the duty to care for his or her own health or to seek such care from others. Those whose task it is to care for the sick must do so conscientiously and admin-

ister the remedies that seem necessary and useful. . . . It is also permitted, with the patient's consent, to interrupt these means, where the results fall short of expectations. . . . When inevitable death is imminent in spite of the means used, it is permitted in conscience to take the decision to refuse forms of treatment that would only secure a precarious and burdensome prolongation of life.[5]

The emphasis is clearly on personal responsibility, exercised within the context of faith in God. Each of us, according to this view, has been given the gift of life from God, and each of us must decide how he or she is going to use God's good gift. Therefore, the privilege of stewardship extends to decisions regarding life-sustaining treatment.

The Roman Catholic Church views decisions regarding medical treatments as life-affirming activity. The gift of life is to be utilized to draw close to God and to experience community with fellow human beings. Death is a part of life that is to be accepted with faith and courage. Treatment decisions affirm all of life—including sickness, suffering, and death—to be different aspects of our journey with God.

Until recently, physicians usually called the shots when it came to treatment decisions. The paternalistic attitude was that the doctor knew best and the patient should follow directions. Now, however, decision making is seen as a collaborative effort. Health care professionals provide the treatment information and emotional support necessary to empower patients to make these personal decisions. Physicians, for example, now need to consider the patients' unique set of values when giving counsel and advice. This holds true for competent as well as noncompetent patients, because the fundamental and abiding right to self-determination in medical treatment decisions extends to a once-competent person who becomes noncompetent.

Self-Determination and Noncompetent Patients Who Have Advance Directives

The President's Commission clearly expressed that a surrogate decision maker can make treatment decisions for a noncompetent patient:

> In most circumstances, patients are presumed to be capable of making decisions about their own care. When a patient's capability to make final decisions is seriously limited, he or she needs to be protected against the adverse consequences of a flawed choice. Yet any mechanism that offers such protection also risks abuse: the individual's ability to direct his or her own life might be frustrated in an unwarranted manner. In its report on informed consent, the Commission recommended that a surrogate—typically a close relative or friend—be named when a patient lacks the capacity to make particular medical decisions.[6]

The "Declaration on Euthanasia" also clearly identifies the patient as the primary decision maker. Patients who lack decision making capacity should have surrogates determine the course of treatment, based on the careful evaluation of information supplied from health care professionals. As the Declaration states: "But for such a decision to be made, account will have to be taken of the reasonable wishes of the patient and the patient's family, as also of the advice of the doctors who are specially competent in the matter."[7]

When a once-competent patient who has written an advance directive loses the ability to make informed decisions, his or her right to self-determination can be upheld in one of two ways: (1) through a designated surrogate decision maker, usually called an "agent," "attorney-in-fact," or a "proxy," or (2) through written instructions detailing personal values and possible treatment choices. When a once-competent individual who has an advance directive becomes noncompetent, treatment decisions should then be made by the designated surrogate or by following the patient's stated instructions.

One important feature of some types of advance directives is a provision that enables a competent person to select a surrogate decision maker prior to losing one's ability to make decisions. Naming a person in advance of serious illness greatly reduces the potential for disagreements among interested parties. Each of us has the right to choose any person we desire to serve as our surrogate decision maker in the event we become unable to make competent medical decisions for ourselves. This is a very personal choice.

Some people, however, will not feel comfortable asking anyone to fulfill this role. These people can then write advance directives that are instructive in nature and describe their preferences and values. When a person writes an instructive advance directive, treatment preferences and personal values must be stated clearly. Otherwise, if he or she becomes noncompetent and treatment options do not match up neatly with his or her stated desires, confusion and uncertainty may result.

Anyone who writes an instructive directive would be wise to have a complete discussion of values and preferences with his or her physician. When these matters have been discussed openly, it is often easier for the physician to make decisions for a noncompetent patient who has not designated a surrogate decision maker in his or her advance directive. One group of physicians has recommended that every advance directive include the following statement for the physician to sign:

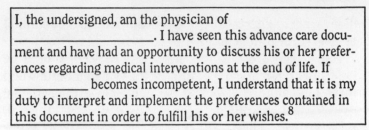

I, the undersigned, am the physician of
_____. I have seen this advance care document and have had an opportunity to discuss his or her preferences regarding medical interventions at the end of life. If
_____ becomes incompetent, I understand that it is my duty to interpret and implement the preferences contained in this document in order to fulfill his or her wishes.[8]

Thus the most important factor in planning for the possibility of future noncompetence is for clear, comprehensive communication to take place between the person who writes the directive and his or her physician and family. To accomplish this, each of us must think through what is important to us and must document our wishes.

A Noncompetent Patient Who Has No Advance Directive

In cases where once-competent people who have no advance directives become noncompetent patients, their family members and/or physicians lack the luxury of written treatment preferences from the patients. However, these patients still have the inherent right to self-determination. In these cases, health care professionals need to exercise great care to ensure that the patients' right to self-determination is protected from those who might hasten their deaths.

Even though these patients have not formally named anyone to make health care decisions for them, health care professionals should seek in each case a surrogate decision maker, preferably a family member or close friend, who can provide guidance in making treatment decisions. From an ethical standpoint, the surrogate should be the person who is in the best position to know the patient's feelings and desires regarding treatment. So a close friend may be parallel or even superior to a family member as a surrogate.

Surrogate decision makers, as we've seen, should be guided by their understanding of the patients' values and preferences. If the surrogates are uncertain of the patients' desires, or if no suitable surrogates are available, then all those people involved—the team of care givers, family members, friends, physicians—will have to carefully consider which treatment options are in the patient's best interest. Choosing treatment that would serve the patient's best interest is the appropriate standard of judgment when specific values and preferences have not been documented.

Making Treatment Decisions

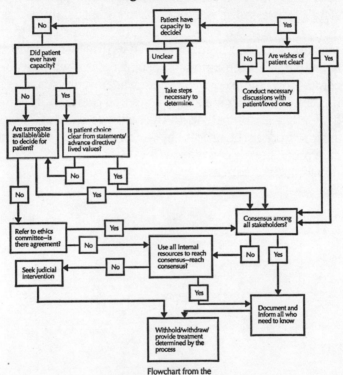

Flowchart from the
Center for Healthcare Ethics
a service of
St. Joseph Health System

Different states have passed laws to help protect non-competent patients placed in difficult treatment situations. As we saw in Chapter 1, some states require "clear and convincing evidence" of a noncompetent patient's previously expressed preferences before life-sustaining treatment is withdrawn or withheld. Other states require that specific treatments be mentioned in writing before they may be withdrawn from a noncompetent patient who was once competent. This prudent protection against abuse shows the importance of documenting values and preferences while a person is still competent. In the next two chapters, we will explore further the process by which surrogates and health care professionals can make ethical treatment decisions for noncompetent patients.

CHAPTER 4

The Sanctity of Life and "Principle of Proportionality"

The sanctity of life plays an important role in life-sustaining treatment decisions. Assisted suicide and active euthanasia are not legal in this country. They are not ethically justifiable, at least not according to mainline Judeo-Christian principles. Ethicists have traditionally made an important distinction between intentionally causing a person's death (i.e., *killing*) and allowing a fatal illness to finish its course. Kevin O'Rourke, a leading Roman Catholic ethicist, describes the distinction this way: "When a person will not benefit from medical care, however, the intention of people removing the care is not to bring about death, but rather to admit that the illness or pathology threatening death cannot be treated in a manner that is beneficial for the patient."[1]

The Hastings Center report, *Guidelines on the Termination of Life-Sustaining Treatment and the Care of the Dying,* explicitly addresses the value commonly referred to as the sanctity of life as it relates to making treatment decisions:

Our society forbids assisting suicide or active euthanasia, even if the motive is compassionate. This prohibition serves to sustain the societal value of respect for life and to provide some safeguards against abuse of the authority to take actions that shorten life. . . . By creating a presumption in favor of continued treatment, the sanctity of life can also help to protect gravely ill patients who are vulnerable. This presumption can reassure society that termination of treatment decisions are being made by individuals, institutions, or by society only after careful scrutiny and justification, and not out of ethically illicit motives.[2]

This principle of the sanctity of life safeguards vulnerable people such as the developmentally disabled who are mentally retarded. The U.S. Supreme Court has affirmed this principle by what it has determined to be immoral, illegal, and unacceptable. The Court did not say we have a right to have someone help us end our lives (assisted suicide) or to have a physician intentionally give medication or treatment that would cause our death (euthanasia). There is an ethical and legal difference between withholding or withdrawing life-sustaining treatment and willfully, knowingly, causing a person's death by assisted suicide or euthanasia.

The Sanctity of Life and Suicide

Much has been written about legalizing physician-assisted suicide for people who are suffering from painful, terminal illnesses. Although none of us would ever want to see a person's suffering increase, it is not in our best interest as a society to make such procedures legal. We must retain the legal and ethical distinction between assisted suicide and withholding or withdrawing a treatment that no longer benefits the patient. There is simply too much potential for abuse when this distinction becomes blurred. Recent developments, such as Dr. Jack Kevorkian's "suicide machines," and Derek Humphry's book, *Final Exit: The Practicalities of Self-Deliverance and Assisted Suicide for the Dying,* confirm that people are increasingly concerned about retaining control over their bodies when serious illness strikes. However, the desire for self-determination can be accomplished through careful communication with physicians and loved ones and by documentation of personal values and preferences in advance directives, not by choosing suicide.

It should never be permissible for health care professionals or surrogates to actively do something with the specific goal of taking a patient's life. We have to admit, though, that the main reason there is presently a move toward assisted suicide is because our present health care system has failed in two important areas: (1) Many people do not have access to the system; and (2) even people who have access are deathly afraid of dying a lonely death in uncontrollable pain. Both of these problems must be addressed.

Instead of legalizing assisted suicide or euthanasia, we should encourage health care professionals to obtain special training in pain management. Studies have shown that in almost all cases, even in cases of bone cancer and other terribly debilitating diseases, pain can be relieved with proper treatment. Yet to date, in our country, we have done a horrible job of pain management. Medical doctors who graduated in June of 1993, for instance, only received an average of 1.9 hours of training in pain control. Only two questions on the oncologist board examination relate to pain.

This lack of training in pain management has contributed to more and more people feeling that assisted suicide is the only answer. The truth is that much of the answer lies in adequate pain management. The "Declaration on Euthanasia" shares this perspective concerning the relief of physical pain:

> At this point it is fitting to recall a declaration by Pius XII, which retains its full force; in answer to a group of doctors who had put the question: "Is the suppression of pain and consciousness by the use of narcotics . . . permitted by religion and morality to the doctor and the patient (even at the approach of death and if one foresees that the use of narcotics will shorten life)?" The Pope said: "If no other means exist, and if, in the given circumstances, this does not prevent the carrying out of other religious and moral duties: Yes." In this case, of course, death is in no way intended or sought, even if the risk of it is reasonably taken; the intention is simply to relieve pain effectively, using for this purpose painkillers available to medicine.[3]

We have to stop telling people to just say no to drugs if they are really sick and need them. People in real pain often need drugs in the form of prescribed medication to alleviate their pain. If we could really put into practice the ideas of compassion and common sense, then more than five hundred thousand people wouldn't have bought *Final Exit*. The solution, as I see it, is to fix the system, not to insist that patients take their own lives because the health care system has its priorities out of sync. We need to intensify our efforts to make euthanasia an unnecessary choice.

As a society, we have a special obligation to protect the elderly and disabled. The elderly often make the most poignant arguments supporting their right to determine the quality of their lives and the time and manner of their deaths. Proponents of assisted suicide begin with the competent, but before you know it the practice includes noncompetent people as well. People all too quickly decide that certain people would be "better off dead." Hitler, for example, convinced the medical community in Nazi Germany that the mentally retarded were "life unworthy of life" and set out to systematically eradicate the "imperfect." We cannot afford to go down that road again.

When a patient will no longer benefit from medical care, the intention of those who seek to remove the treatment in question should be to admit that the illness will be fatal and/or that prolonging treatment will be either futile, torturous, or inordinately burdensome *for the patient*. This is not a desire to cause the patient's death; it is a decision not to torment or burden the patient inordinately. When life-sustaining treatment is withheld or withdrawn in a case of severe or overwhelming illness, we are recognizing the limits of medical technology and accepting death as the natural, final stage of earthly life.

Understanding the Sanctity of Life and Proportionality

The Hastings Center's *Guidelines on the Termination of Life-Sustaining Treatment and the Care of the Dying* clearly acknowledges the value and sanctity of life, prohibits assisted suicide and euthanasia, and respects the self-determination of the patient and the patient's surrogate to make treatment decisions. Recognizing the sanctity of both life and death leads us toward the principle of proportionality in medical treatment, which serves as a valuable guideline in making treatment decisions, particularly when surrogates or health care providers must make those decisions for others.

Because the proper goal of medicine is to promote the patient's well-being, which involves identifying the benefits and burdens of the treatment from the patient's perspective and deciding what is in the patient's best interest, the well-being of the patient is a dominant theme in the Hastings Center report. The report properly places the patient's well-being within the context of relationships in which a person is involved at the time of an illness. These relationships place the patient at the hub of a wheel, with spokes reaching out to connect him or her to a community of people. Therefore, everyone involved—health care professionals and significant others—should work to empower the patient and implement his or her decisions regarding treatment.[4]

The Roman Catholic Church's pronouncements on the morality of medical treatments are strikingly similar to these guidelines. In addition, Roman Catholic and other religious traditions strongly reflect a basic belief in the intrinsic value of human life and, therefore, add a theological perspective to the principle of proportionality.

This theological perspective enhances the principle of proportionality by focusing our attention on the Giver and the gift of life. All living creatures, including disabled human beings, are good gifts from God to be celebrated and cared for with respect. God endows each of us with blessings that make us unique. Remembering the gift of life and the Giver of life expands the principle of proportionality so that we strive for treatments which not only benefit a patient but help celebrate each patient as a unique child of God.

According to this viewpoint, all human life is seen as part of God's good creation. Human lives are, therefore, bound to the living God of the universe by the power of God's love, which created the world from nothing and sustains every living creature. This deeply-held regard for the gift of life does not mean that all available means of medical technology must be utilized at all times to preserve physical life. Mere physical life is not an absolute value. Life has value and meaning only insofar as a person is able to have relationships with other people and with God. In other words, life is meaningful to the extent that a person is able to pursue the spiritual ends of human life.

The Roman Catholic Church places primary importance on the principle of proportionality. Richard McCormick, a professor of Christian ethics, has expressed it this way:

> What Pius XII was saying, then, is that forcing (morally) one to take *all* means [of medical treatment] is tantamount to forcing attention and energies on a subordinate good in a way that prejudices a higher good, even eventually making it unrecognizable as a good. Excessive concern for the temporal is at some point neglect of the eternal. An obligation to use all means to preserve life would be a devaluation of human life, since it would remove life from the context or story that is the source of its ultimate value.[5]

The approach is clear: The benefits of any life-sustaining treatment must justify the imposed burdens. The benefits must be sufficient to enable the individual to pursue the ultimate goal of life—fellowship with God and with the human family. Pope John Paul II agreed with this viewpoint: "When inevitable death is imminent in spite of the means used, it is permitted in conscience to take the decision to refuse forms of treatment that would only secure a precarious and burdensome prolongation of life."[6]

An important aspect of the "Declaration on Euthanasia" is its treatment of death. The document points out the need for balance. It advocates an ethical position that acknowledges the sanctity of all human life while at the same time explicitly stating that within Christian theology there is a sanctity of death ethic as well:

Today it is very important to protect, at the moment of death, both the dignity of the human person and the Christian concept of life, against a technological attitude that threatens to become an abuse. Thus some people speak of a "right to die," which is an expression that does not mean the right to procure death either by one's own hand or by means of someone else, as one pleases, but rather the right to die peacefully with human and Christian dignity.... Life is a gift of God, and on the other hand death is unavoidable; it is necessary, therefore, that we, without in any way hastening the hour of death, should be able to accept it with full responsibility and dignity.[7]

This statement provides a framework for an understanding of life and death that protects the dignity of both. Each human life is valued regardless of handicap, and death is acknowledged as the natural end of earthly existence. Death is, therefore, accepted as part of life, not something to be avoided at all costs. Death is not seen as the final illness that technology will someday overcome.

The lasting contribution of Roman Catholic moral theology concerning treatment decisions rests on these two principles: the sanctity of both life and death as gifts from God, and the principle of proportionality (the weighing of the benefits and burdens of treatment from the patient's perspective).

The Roman Catholic Church does not stand alone in this viewpoint. A wide range of religious communities in our country have stated the principles of sanctity of life and proportionality in similar ways. These statements focus attention on the individual's relationship to God, to family, to friends, and to the created order. They emphasize that when a person loses the capacity to maintain meaningful relationships, or if mere physical life is being maintained by medical technology, then it is permissible to limit life-sustaining treatment.

It is clear from these religious perspectives that all available means of treatment do not have to be used if such treatment does not benefit the patient. The consensus of a variety of religious perspectives is to do what can be done to produce a cure or make the patient comfortable, but not to use medical technology solely to prolong an inevitable death. For example, let's consider the following perspective of the Presbyterian Church (USA):

> While the direction of biblical ethics is against taking the life of another, it in no way claims that it is necessary to prolong the life—or the dying process—of a person who is gravely ill with little or no hope for cure or remission. Persons who are terminally ill must be able to trust that their dying will not be prolonged by unrequested technological interventions.... Whatever its origin, ambivalence is woven into the fabric of being itself, and decisions of life and death are met with a kind of frustrating ambiguity. Since life-death situations can rarely be made with certainty, even when all the evidence is in, decisions must be made with humility and with a posture of seeking God's forgiveness and acceptance."[8]

In order for a medical treatment to be ethically mandatory, then, the benefits of treatment must outweigh the burdens as measured by the total well-being of the patient. If the benefits don't outweigh the burdens, it is ethically acceptable to withhold or withdraw the treatment. When that treatment provides more benefits than burdens from the patient's perspective, it should be provided. When it is unclear whether the burdens or benefits are greater, it is appropriate to err on the side of life and provide treatment. For example, if a proposed course of treatment would be extremely painful or intrusive, it would still be proportionate if the prognosis were for a complete cure or at least significant improvement in the patient's condition. On the other hand, a treatment course that is only minimally painful or intrusive may nonetheless be considered disproportionate to the potential benefits if the patient's prognosis involves virtually no significant improvement.

Proportionality and Futile Treatment

Applying the principles of sanctity of life and proportionality to bioethical dilemmas can greatly enhance our ability to begin to address difficult issues such as futile treatment with a sense of justice and equity. Based on the principle of proportionality, futile treatment can be defined as any treatment that will likely not provide, in the judgment of the patient and/or the physician, a notable improvement for the patient. Thereby, futile treatment imposes a greater burden than benefit on a particular patient at a specific time in the patient's history. However, health care providers must often make treatment decisions without the benefit of knowing for certain that the treatment will work. This has led to ethical discussions on medical futility, as people try to determine when a treatment should be provided and when providing it is futile and will provide little, if any, benefit.

One difficulty in making treatment decisions occurs when a competent patient or the noncompetent patient's surrogate asks for, or in some cases demands, treatment that a physician considers to be futile. For example, one woman's family felt that a hospital should continue tube feedings for her even though she was eighty-five years old, had had a series of strokes that permanently damaged her brain, and was diagnosed as being in a persistent vegetative state in which she had no conscious awareness. The hospital felt that continued treatment was futile because she would never regain an awareness of her surroundings. Many people viewed the family's demand for all possible medical interventions as unreasonable because no medical treatment could provide a net gain for this patient.

Futility is a difficult issue. It goes to the heart of the patient-physician relationship. Patients, as we've seen, possess a basic right to self-determination. But at the same time, physicians have a professional responsibility to act according to their values and sense of integrity. So self-determination must be balanced in the light of the sanctity of life and the issue of proportionality. Some ethicists would argue that it is not ethically acceptable for a patient to ask health care professionals to provide treatment that would violate these two principles. Some would argue that physicians are not obligated to provide treatment that provides no reasonable expectation of improvement in the patient's condition. Others have gone so far as to say that physicians are not obligated to provide any medical treatment that simply preserves permanent unconsciousness or does not eliminate dependence on intensive medical care.

In an effort to resolve the questions raised when futile treatment is requested, Daniel Callahan of the Hastings Center advocates an approach that would seek a social mechanism to reach mutually agreed-upon standards. This would resolve the tension by recognizing both the patients' and the physicians' integrity through general standards that could be applied when making value judgments. Callahan poses the following thought-provoking questions:

> If our need is to avoid death, must medicine give us immortality to achieve that need? If our need is to avoid sickness, does this entail a societal obligation to find a way

to bring health to, say, a 400-gram baby, a baby who cannot now survive but might if we invest a few million dollars to make that possible? Is there a medical need to save each and every baby, no matter how small and how immature, assuming a technically feasible means could be found for doing so? Would the "need" to triumph over death-dealing disease justify an artificial heart for someone aged 100 suffering from heart disease?[9]

These difficult and emotionally laden questions will not be answered easily. We need to pursue moral principles that will help us address the complexity of these problems. In seeking to understand the limits of medical technology, we need to think collectively of the common good. We need to determine which policies and strategies will allow the greatest number of people to live with basic human dignity. We need to move beyond the self-centered "What I want for me and my family" to the more community-minded "With limited resources and limited capabilities of medical technology, what should we seek for the common good?" At some point, patient self-determination must be balanced with respect for the responsibilities of health care professionals and a desire to serve the common good. Achieving this balance will make us consider the societal values we wish to pursue and will give us a structure by which we can resolve situations in which values clash.

CHAPTER 5

Unresolved Ethical Issues

Although our society has made significant progress during the past two decades, it has not resolved a number of procedural issues related to the administration of medical treatment in certain cases. We have (except for rare cases when futile treatment is demanded) determined that any competent person can make his or her own treatment decisions. We have determined that a competent person can document his or her treatment preferences so that those preferences will be honored should he or she become noncompetent. We also have a sufficiently universal consensus on the principles of the sanctity of life and proportionality, which serves as a valid guideline for making less clear-cut ethical judgments on medical treatment decisions. However, we still face many difficult, sometimes controversial, questions when we make treatment decisions for noncompetent patients who have never been competent, individuals in persistent vegetative state, and patients who need artificial nutrition and hydration. Let's now consider the reality of delivering treatment in these delicate situations.

Patients Who Have Never Been Competent

A number of procedural issues related to noncompetent patients and their abiding right to accept or refuse medical treatment remain unresolved: Who speaks for the patient who has never been competent? What if the patient has never expressed views on the subject? Or what if the patient has been noncompetent since birth? As a "reliable person," may a guardian substitute his or her values and judgment and attempt to determine the patient's best interest?

Severely ill newborns and some mentally retarded persons constitute a unique group of people who have never been competent to make informed decisions regarding their medical care. In all cases of severely ill newborns, and in many cases of persons with mental retardation, their values or desires cannot be known. Although these individuals have the right to self-determination, they are effectively unable to personally exercise this right. Furthermore, these patients are unable to formulate advance directives, and their surrogates cannot make decisions based on previously discussed values.

At times, questions concerning life-sustaining treatment for these noncompetent patients will arise. We must take extreme care to make proper ethical decisions in these very difficult cases. It is imperative that we, as a society, protect fragile and vulnerable patients who have often been devalued because of their handicapping conditions. We must have a societal commitment to care for those who are the weakest.

All those whose situations involve noncompetent patients should seek to discover what is in the overall best interest of each patient, even in the midst of the uncertainties that go along with medical decision making. An appropriate medical decision reflects the patient's best interest, balancing the burdens and benefits of each proposed medical treatment. If these principles are followed, decision making will be consistent for noncompetent patients who have no advance directives.

Parents are usually the preferred surrogates who are asked to make treatment decisions regarding critically-ill newborns. Public policy should not invade family decision making unless there is clear and convincing evidence that parents are acting against the best interests of their children. Obviously parents must consent to procedures that are clearly beneficial to their children.

In cases where it is unclear whether treatment is more of a benefit than a burden, complete and accurate medical information must be presented, and the medical community needs to provide emotional support for surrogate decision makers. Most often in these cases, decision making will be a process that takes time in order for those involved to fully assess the effectiveness of the options. These cases require ongoing honest and open communication between surrogates and health care professionals, which must be carefully documented and monitored through quality assurance procedures.

All those who make decisions on behalf of noncompetent patients should weigh the benefits and burdens of treatment and seek to act in the patients' best interests. In order to decide what is in a patient's best interest, we must consider the many factors that comprise the patient's personal identity. Each of us has a unique set of priorities and preferences, all of which should be considered when we determine what is in a patient's best interest. Basically this amounts to evaluating the overall framework of each patient's relationships and then determining whether a given treatment will enhance the patient's ability to pursue personal values at that time.

This "best interest of the patient" standard is what the

courts have determined to be most useful when ruling on these types of cases. William A. Karis, an attorney experienced in developmentally disabled-related issues, writes:

> The best test requires the court to consider the actual best interests of a developmentally disabled person, and not the interests of others or the general public. The test does not, however, require the court to know what the mentally disabled patient views as her best interests. The standard is an objective one. Finally, this test recognizes that the incompetent developmentally disabled person's right to choose whether to terminate treatment cannot be effectively exercised. The best interest test is the most feasible way to protect this right.[1]

Cases which involve people who have never been competent to make medical treatment decisions and who have no available surrogate decision makers are some of the most difficult in medical ethics. Cautious, principled discussion must take place before any life-sustaining treatment is withheld or withdrawn. These decisions should involve a careful determination of the benefits and burdens of the life-sustaining treatment and should focus on each patient's overall well-being. Here, more than with any other group of patients, it is important to err on the side of continued treatment. Their rights must be protected by careful, case-by-case decision making.

Great care must be taken, for example, to protect the rights of adult persons with mental retardation who have no family members actively involved in their lives. When questions concerning life-sustaining treatment for these individuals arise, these decisions should be made by an interdisciplinary ethics committee whose membership includes a patients' rights advocate and a wide cross-section of health care professionals. All such discussions must be properly documented and should be reviewed regularly.

Under a pilot program established by the New York State legislature, volunteer committees may be empowered to make decisions about medical care in cases involving noncompetent patients who have no available surrogates. A law protects physicians from liability when they rely on the committees' decisions. After some time, this method has proven effective in producing quick, careful, and individualized decisions. The program has circumvented the time-consuming, costly approach of petitioning for a court-appointed guardian for each patient who lacks decision-making capacity and has no appropriate surrogate.[2]

Persistent Vegetative State

Approximately ten thousand patients who live in various types of treatment centers in the United States are in a persistent vegetative state. *Persistent vegetative state* refers to a condition in which the upper portion of the brain, the cerebral cortex, is permanently and irreparably damaged. This portion of the brain is responsible for conscious thought and self-awareness. It is the part that enables us to think about ourselves. Patients whose cerebral cortexes have suffered verifiable and permanent damage can have a variety of reflexive responses but have no conscious awareness and do not feel pain. They have lost the capacity to have relationships with other people. These tragic situations are extremely difficult for everyone involved.

When patients have been accurately diagnosed as being in a persistent vegetative state, there is no possibility that they will recover cognitive awareness. They will never again be "connected" to reality as we know it. They will remain in a vegetative "twilight zone." They can "live" in such a condition because the brain stem—the lower portion of the brain that controls autonomic functions such as respiration and circulation—is often completely intact and functioning properly. People in a persistent vegetative state may breathe on their own but must have artificially supplied nutrition and hydration (tube feeding) because they are unable to swallow. That is why the court stated that Nancy Beth Cruzan was "oblivious to her environment." She remained in a persistent vegetative state from 1983 until she died on December 26, 1990.

These patients present a great challenge. Some people have advocated that the definition of brain death should be expanded to include these patients. "Carefully test to verify the diagnosis of PVS," they say, "then suspend all life-sustaining treatment and allow the patients to be pronounced dead." Others argue, "People in PVS are the most fragile of all patients. They should, therefore, be strongly protected and treated aggressively." Some state courts have ruled that any treatment for a person in PVS is considered to be too much treatment and therefore a burden to the patient because there is no possibility of recovery.[3] Other states require special documentation before artificial nutrition and hydration can be removed from a patient in PVS.

No workable consensus has yet emerged concerning PVS patients. There is no easy answer; every answer is filled with strong emotions. In considering treatment decisions for patients in PVS, health care professionals, religious professionals, and society as a whole must proceed cautiously lest we hastily and carelessly pronounce people "dead." History shows that once these discussions begin, the mentally retarded are too quickly added to the list, along with others whom society views as "expendable." Any consensus on treatment for these patients must be narrowly defined. Their diagnosis must be verified over a substantial period of time, and their life-sustaining treatment should be withdrawn only upon the request of concerned family members or surrogates.

Pondering the best interest of patients in PVS will force us to consider what we consider the goals and limits of medical technology. It will force us to wrestle with our collective values. Someone once said that the way a society treats its weakest members is the clearest indication of the true nature of that society. We must consider this issue because, as medical technology advances, our ability to sustain "life" in a persistent vegetative state will increase.

Artificial Nutrition and Hydration

During the past few years, the treatment that has sparked the most heated debate is the artificial provision of nutrition and hydration (tube feeding), especially when it is provided to people who are in a persistent vegetative state. Some cities and communities consider the issue of whether to provide or withhold artificial nutrition and hydration to be ongoing. Some guidelines, such as those developed by the Joint Committee on Bioethics of the San Diego County Medical Society and San Diego County Bar Association, recognize that this medical treatment should be open to discussion.

> Foregoing hydration and nutrition has historically been controversial and evokes emotional responses because of the symbolic value of maintaining basic food and fluids. . . . However, it is now widely accepted that they [artificial nutrition and hydration] may be considered similar to other life-sustaining treatments.[4]

A number of court rulings related to artificial nutrition and hydration have considered this treatment to be similar to any other life-sustaining medical treatment. In response, some communities in the United States have moved to consider all life-sustaining treatments to be similar. Consider the following guidelines developed by the Joint Committee on Bioethics, Los Angeles County Medical Association, and Los Angeles County Bar Association:

> Medically administered nutrition and hydration (i.e., including NG [nasogastric] tubes, gastrostomies, intravenously administered fluids, and hyperalimentation) should be analyzed in the same way as any other medical treatment. Nutrition and hydration have a powerful symbolic significance to many members of the public, as well as to many caregivers. It is therefore particularly important that those people who take care of the patient fully understand the rationale for any order to forgo medically administered nutrition and hydration.[5]

In cases of permanent coma and/or persistent vegetative state, some courts have repeatedly stated that any and all medical treatment may be stopped at the request of the surrogate decision maker.[6] In an important article in *The New England Journal of Medicine*, Drs. Steinbrook and Lo address this approach to the withholding or withdrawal of artificial nutrition and hydration:

> These developments suggest an emerging medical, ethical, and legal consensus on the situations in which artificial feeding can be withdrawn. The focus of the discussion should be the patient's wishes, not the type of treatment or the patient's prognosis. Artificial feeding can be viewed on a level with other medical interventions—cardiopulmonary resuscitation, mechanical ventilation, dialysis,

antibiotic therapy. It should not be considered a part of "ordinary care" or the routine provision of nursing care and comfort. Competent patients have the right to refuse this treatment after assessing for themselves the benefits and burdens. This right is not limited to comatose or terminally ill patients. For incompetent patients, feeding, like other treatments, can be stopped in accordance with the patient's previously expressed wishes.[7]

While it can be said that for the most part there is legal and medical agreement on the issue of withholding or withdrawing artificial nutrition and hydration, we do not find the same level of agreement within the Roman Catholic tradition.

Although the question of artificial nutrition and hydration has moved to the forefront of ethical debate during the past five years, Catholics addressed this issue more than thirty years ago. This discussion of artificial nutrition and hydration has focused on the principle of proportionality: what provides an overall benefit for the patient. Some people feel that if a person is not able to take food by normal means (through the mouth with the ability to swallow) then the medical treatment of artificial feeding does not necessarily benefit the patient. Others feel that the symbolic nature of providing food and water—the two elements necessary to sustain life—is an overriding factor that would mandate tube feeding for all persons—even those in a persistent vegetative state.

Kevin O'Rourke has clarified the position of Catholics who take the position that it is ethically justifiable to withhold or withdraw artificial nutrition and hydration. He writes:

Withholding artificial hydration and nutrition from a patient in an irreversible coma . . . allows an already fatal pathology to take its natural course. . . . One of the basic ethical assumptions upon which medicine and efforts to nurse and feed people are based is that life should be prolonged because living enables us to pursue the purpose of life. . . . If efforts to prolong life are useless or result in a severe burden for the patient insofar as the pursuing the purpose of life is concerned, then the ethical obligation to prolong life is no longer present.[8]

A number of Roman Catholics, however, disagree with this interpretation. Robert Barry, in an article entitled "Feeding the Comatose and the Common Good in the Catholic Tradition," traces the history of Roman Catholic moral theology on this subject. He concludes that withdrawing artificially supplied nutrition and hydration is killing by omission.

Food and water, irrespective of their mode of provision, are basic resources of the body and are not therapeutic measures. . . . Unlike medical treatments, all people require them whether they are well or ill. To remove them when their mere provision is by routine techniques of patient maintenance is to kill the patient by omission through their denial. Removing them does not allow an underlying pathological condition to be set free, but sets the process of dying immediately into motion.[9]

Barry argues that moral theologian Francisco Vitoria states that we have a moral obligation to give and receive only the customarily and commonly available forms of care and feeding in a society. He goes on to say that Vitoria maintained that taking food is not obligatory if great effort is required (meaning great effort on the part of the ill patient).

From these statements, Barry concludes that tube feedings in our day constitute "common" forms of taking food. Others would argue that feeding by a nasogastric or gastrostomy tube is an "uncommon" means of taking nutrition.

Clearly the issue of withholding and withdrawing artificial nutrition and hydration is difficult to resolve because of the symbolic significance of food and water. Many people believe this treatment should be evaluated in the same manner as any other medical treatment. Others believe we should draw the line here because of the symbolic significance of food and water. Still others believe it is never morally acceptable to withhold or withdraw artificial nutrition and hydration, even from a patient in PVS. Some would apply the principle of proportionality to this treatment, asking if the provision of this treatment provides any new benefit for the patient.

> With regard to medical interventions—whether medicinal, surgical, or mechanical—withholding or discontinuing them becomes ethical when they involve what one perceives to be grave burdens on oneself or others, according to the circumstances of person, place, time, and culture. . . . What is ethically more important for the patient is not the medical outcome of using or not using these procedures but their burdensomeness in terms of the physical, economic, psychological, or spiritual factors involved.[10]

Thus, the issue of withholding or withdrawing artificially supplied nutrition and hydration remains controversial. It presents an extremely difficult challenge for level-of-care staff who provide hands-on treatment to patients who receive artificial nutrition and hydration. The bond that forms between these workers and their patients is very strong.

Although there are no easy answers, I propose that any decisions to limit such life-sustaining treatment should include the input of the treatment staff as well as the input of an available surrogate. Such decisions should also be made over a period of time in order to give everyone involved the opportunity to "grow into" the decision and feel comfortable with the process involved. We need to work toward the development of a workable consensus for patients who don't have available surrogates, for patients in persistent vegetative state, and for the provision of artificial nutrition and hydration. How we seek to resolve these dilemmas speaks volumes about the values we deem essential to our society.

CHAPTER 6

"Advance Directives" for Informed Consent

During the past twenty-five years, there has been rapid change in health care and our attitudes toward it. Americans are thinking more about their health care and are becoming more educated about health-related issues. Many have concluded that it is in their best interest to take a more active role in their medical treatment decisions.

As we've seen, the intent of The Patient Self-Determination Act of 1990 is to guarantee every patient the opportunity to document his or her treatment preferences. This is accomplished through an advance directive, which extends the principle of self-determination once a patient is no longer capable of making informed choices. Because advance directives are the key to making our desires known concerning life-sustaining medical treatments, it's important for each of us to think about our personal values and to write some form of advance directive.

Advance directives have been used since 1969, when the Living Will first appeared on the scene. Since then, each of the fifty states have passed some type of legislation concerning advance directives. Recent court rulings have indicated that all people have the right to formalize advance directives. Although advance directives do have limits, they are useful tools when executed properly and when shared with each patient's health care team.

Despite widespread agreement that every competent adult should execute an advance directive, they are used infrequently. In 1987, only 9 percent of Americans had written advance directives for medical care. Since then, we have made little headway. Today most adults in the United States still do not have an advance directive for medical care. The lack of advance directives is further complicated by the fact that even when patients have executed directives, their physicians often do not know about them.

Clearly, an immense amount of work lies before health care professionals, religious professionals, and others who are in a position to encourage and assist individuals in preparing advance directives. But there is hope for significant progress. Consider the results of a 1988 study conducted at Massachusetts General Hospital in Boston to determine the population's awareness of and willingness to write an advance directive. Ninety-four percent of those who participated in the fourteen-minute survey and who were less than sixty-five years old and in good to excellent health wanted to discuss an advance directive with their physicians and execute such a document. The surveyors used a questionnaire that outlined possible medical treatment scenarios. When the interviewers asked people to imagine themselves noncompetent with a poor prognosis, the individuals questioned decided against life-sustaining treatment about 70 percent of the time.

The results of this study are clear: People want to be educated about their rights and the issues, and to write the advance directives of their choice. In fact, the overwhelming majority of people interviewed wanted to execute advance directives. However, desire alone is insufficient to motivate people to complete an advance directive.

Why Don't People Write Advance Directives?

Although we know that each of us will die one day, facing the reality of death when we are healthy is not easy. So the greatest challenge of The Patient Self-Determination Act of 1990 lies in the fact that most people feel uncomfortable discussing the issues that surround serious illness, suffering, dying, and death. Even physicians do not like to discuss death and dying; they are trained to view death as the enemy that must be defeated.

Our reluctance to discuss these issues is part of the human condition. Ernest Becker, a Pulitzer Prize-winning author, is correct. People spend most of their time and energy denying the central truth of the human condition: Every person will die sooner or later. He writes:

> I don't believe that the complex symbol of death is ever absent, no matter how much vitality and inner sustainment a person has. . . . Man is literally split in two: he has an awareness of his own splendid uniqueness in that he sticks out of nature with a towering majesty, and yet he goes back into the ground a few feet in order blindly and dumbly to rot and disappear forever. It is a terrifying dilemma to be in and to have to live with.[1]

Despite our desire to escape death's reality, it is important for all of us to make decisions concerning life-sustaining treatment when we are healthy. By documenting our desires ahead of time, we can avoid much of the stress we and our families face when decisions on life-sustaining treatment must be made. So how can people be encouraged to learn about and execute advance directives? Who should talk with patients about writing advance directives?

Who Can Encourage People to Write Advance Directives?

For most people, physicians are the obvious choice for initiating discussion on a directive. Evidence shows that people don't mind imagining themselves in poor health for the purpose of writing advance directives as long as their physicians initiate the communication process. In fact, one of the most frequently cited barriers to writing an advance directive is the patient's expectation that the physician should initiate such a discussion. Physicians need to take the time to discuss advance directives with their patients. However, all of us, as health care consumers, need to force the issue and initiate such discussions with our physicians. We cannot expect physicians to assume the burden of initiating discussion of advance directives on their own. Physicians, too, are human and have the same reluctance as their patients to talk about the reality of human mortality.

The following poem, written by a physician, captures the essence of the uneasiness most of us feel when thinking about our own deaths:

How Will I Die?

I have often wondered—
How should I die?

Should it be gently
As in a return
To my mother's arms?

Or will it be
With rage, and will
I fight bitterly
Against that which
I know nothing of?

Or will I
Embrace deep darkness—
Battered and broken—
In sudden, head-on, crushing
Collision?

Or will I—
My body a ballroom
For an anarchic diastral dance—
Surface from opium haze, and plead
Please read my living will.

Or will I,
unknowing recipient
Of "life-extending" ingenuity,
Voicelessly shout—let me go—
From endless gray to total dark?

Or should I
With my last breath,
Murmur platitudes
That might make my
Survivors happy?

Or should I
Cry to myself—
I should have gone
To church

Oftener?
Or should I
Smile, and wonder—
At the memorial service,
Will they say good things
Of me?

Solemnly?[2]

Dr. Benson's poem captures a key element of the human condition. We ponder what the end of our lives will be like, but not for too long because a part of us cannot bear to consider our mortality. Yet it's certain that each of us will die. Not one of us knows the day or the hour. Since scientists cannot know the exact day, hour, and minute that an earthquake will occur, the only prudent course of action is to always be as prepared as possible. Being prepared for an earthquake means having extra water, food, a battery-powered radio, and other essentials. Likewise, we do not know when a serious accident or illness which leads to death will strike. Being prepared means documenting our personal values through an advance directive.

We should not assume that physicians alone must initiate discussions concerning advance directives. Any health care professional—physician, nurse, chaplain, social worker, or psychologist—who has an understanding of the issues and a willingness to help people clarify their own personal values can easily be trained to help people complete this important task. These professionals should take time to become familiar with the issues surrounding advance directives and write them for themselves. (It is always easier to discuss issues and values if you can draw on personal experience.)

Religious leaders can also be a valuable resource, providing encouragement and assistance to individuals who are preparing advance directives. Virtually every religious leader has been, or will be, asked to give guidance to a person who is confronting treatment issues or to counsel the loved ones of someone who is. Therefore, religious leaders should take time to become familiar with the issues surrounding life-sustaining treatment and advance directives. Religious professionals who take the lead by considering these issues on a personal level and writing their own advance directives will be better prepared to give guidance to people who have questions than those who haven't addressed these issues on a personal level.

We must also remember that religious institutions can be ideal settings for discussions relating to life-sustaining issues. Within these religious institutions, people can discuss their personal values and issues regarding sickness, suffering, and death in a context that potentially provides more understanding than purely secular institutions.

Regardless of who initiates discussion on treatment decisions and advance directives, the emerging consensus and court decisions are clear on one point: Decisions to limit life-sustaining treatment are personal-value decisions made by competent individuals after they evaluate relevant medical information. All of us live by a set of values, whether we articulate these values in a formal way or not. The difficulty is that virtually all of us need assistance in clarifying our personal-value systems. So the challenge facing health care professionals, religious professionals, and people concerned about the issues of life-sustaining treatment is to provide a context in which people can discuss these serious issues in nonthreatening ways that empower people to take control of the medical decisions that affect their lives and the lives of others.

CHAPTER 7

How to Decide: Advance Directives

Who Should Document Values and Why?

If we each clarify our values and put them in an advance directive while we still have the ability to make informed choices, it will be easier for the surrogate(s) to carry out our wishes if needed. Young people, as well as older people, should discuss these issues and make their desires and preferences known. Often some of the most difficult medical decisions must be made on behalf of younger patients. If young people talk with their family members and friends before a medical crisis arises, those who must make medical treatment decisions for them during a medical crisis can be certain they are following the patients' wishes.

Previous discussion of values and treatment preferences can provide a solid base for families, friends, physicians, and others who may be required to make difficult medical decisions. Furthermore, talking about such issues ahead of time may minimize family disagreements, and when such decisions do need to be made, the decision makers' burden of responsibility may be lessened because they feel confident of the patient's preferences. In the remainder of this chapter, we will examine some of the values that come into play when people make decisions to limit life-sustaining treatment. We'll also consider ways in which we can each clarify and solidify our personal values in order to write a useful advance directive which documents those values.

How to Document Your Values

In documenting your preferences, it is important to let your personal values be your guide. Consider which values are important to you. For example, which of the following statements express how you would feel if you were seriously ill?

My values say it is important for me to:

1. Die without having my life prolonged by machines.
2. Not be a burden to my family.
3. Act according to my religious beliefs.
4. Avoid unnecessary pain and suffering.
5. Make my own decisions as long as I am able to do so.

In addition, we should consider how much life-sustaining intervention we would want. How, for example, would we like the following common interventions to be used if we were unable to make competent decisions concerning our medical treatment?

- Cardiopulmonary resuscitation (CPR) to restore breathing and heartbeat

- Mechanical respiration (ventilator, respirator)
- Intravenous fluids
- Artificial nutrition
- Blood transfusions
- Antibiotic therapy
- Dialysis
- Surgical intervention

Some people advocate the use of a written values history as a way to enhance the effectiveness of an advance directive. In this chapter, we'll look at two ways by which you can clarify your values and medical preferences using the Values History Form and the Medical Directive. By supplementing your advance directive with this type of well-documented information, you will take much of the guesswork out of treatment decisions in the event you become unable to make your own health care treatment decisions.

Your Values History Form

The following Values History Form and the introductory explanation (which I've changed a bit to fit the format of this book) were developed by a team at the University of New Mexico Center for Health Law and Ethics. Although the form is not a legal document, it may be used to supplement your advance directive. The creators of this Values History Form invite readers to use and make copies of the form as needed without concern for copyright violation.

How Do I Fill Out the Values History Form?

In the first section of the form, write down any written or oral instructions you have already prepared. If you have not yet discussed these issues with the appropriate person(s) or written down your preferences, you may choose to complete this section later, perhaps after you have completed Section 2 of the form.

Section 2 asks a number of questions about such issues as your attitude toward your health; your feelings about your health care providers; your thoughts about independence and control; your personal relationships; your overall attitude toward life, including illness and death; your religious background and beliefs; your living environment; your attitude toward finances; and your wishes concerning your funeral.

You can begin to answer these questions in a variety of ways. Perhaps you would like to write out your own thoughts before talking over these questions with someone else. Or you might ask friends and family members to come together and discuss these questions with you. Feel free to add your own questions and comments to those already provided. Remember, it is easier to talk about these issues *before* a medical crisis occurs. As you complete the form, reflect on how you want to live until you die rather than on how you want to die.

What Should I Do with My Completed Values History Form?

Be sure that those who might be involved in making future medical decisions on your behalf—family members, friends, health care providers, lawyers, pastors, and so on—

are aware of your medical treatment desires and preferences. If appropriate, give each of them a copy of your completed Values History Form. Remember, however, that all of us continue to learn and change, so discuss and/or update your Values History regularly as your preferences and values change. Consider attaching a copy of the Values History Form to your advance directive, if you have one. If you don't, file the Values History Form with your important medical papers.

VALUES HISTORY FORM

NAME _____

DATE _____

If someone assisted you in completing this form, please fill in his or her name, address, and relationship to you.

Name   _____

Address   _____

                _____

Relationship   _____

The purpose of this form is to assist you in thinking about and writing down what is important to you about your health. If you should at some time become unable to make health care decisions for yourself, your thoughts as expressed on this form may help others make a decision for you in accordance with what you have chosen.

The first section of this form asks whether you have already expressed your wishes concerning medical treatment through either written or oral communications and if not, whether you would like to do so now. The second section of this form provides an opportunity for you to discuss your values, wishes, and preferences in a number of different areas, such as your personal relationships, your overall attitude toward life, and your thoughts about illness.

SECTION 1

A. WRITTEN LEGAL DOCUMENTS

Have you written any of the following legal documents?

_____

If so, please complete the requested information.

Living Will
Date written: _____

Document location:_____

Comments: (e.g., any limitations, special requests, etc.)

_____

Durable Power of Attorney
Date written: _____

Document location:_____

Comments: (e.g., whom have you named to be your decision maker?)

Durable Power of Attorney for Health Care Decisions
Date written: _____

Document location:_____

Comments: (e.g., whom have you named to be your decision maker?)_____

_____

Organ Donations
Date written: _____

Document location:_____

Comments: (e.g., any limitations on which organs you would like to donate?)_____

_____

B. WISHES CONCERNING SPECIFIC MEDICAL PROCEDURES

If you have ever expressed your wishes, either written or orally, concerning any of the following medical procedures, please complete the requested information. If you have not previously indicated your wishes on these procedures and would like to do so now, please complete this information.

Organ Donation
To whom expressed:_____

If oral, when? _____

If written, when? _____

Document location:_____

Comments:_____

_____

Kidney Dialysis
To whom expressed:_____

If oral, when?_____

If written, when?_____

Document location:_____

Comments:_____

_____

Cardiopulmonary Resuscitation (CPR)
To whom expressed:_____

If oral, when?_____

If written, when?_____

Document location: _____

Comments:_____

_____

Respirators
To whom expressed:_____

If oral, when?_____

If written, when?_____

Document location:_____

Comments:_____

_____

Artificial Nutrition
To whom expressed:

If oral, when?_____

If written, when?_____

Document location:_____

Comments:_____
_____

Artificial Hydration
To whom expressed:_____

If oral, when?_____

If written, when?_____

Document location:_____

Comments:_____
_____

C. GENERAL COMMENTS

Do you wish to make any general comments about the information you provided in this section?
_____
_____

SECTION 2

A. YOUR OVERALL ATTITUDE TOWARD YOUR HEALTH

1. How would you describe your current health status? If you currently have any medical problems, how would you describe them?_____
_____

2. If you have current medical problems, in what ways, if any, do they affect your ability to function?_____
_____

3. How do you feel about your current health status?_____
_____

4. How well are you able to meet the basic necessities of life—eating, food preparation, sleeping, personal hygiene, etc.?_____
_____

5. Do you wish to make any general comments about your overall health?_____
_____
_____
_____

B. YOUR PERCEPTION OF THE ROLE OF YOUR DOCTOR AND OTHER HEALTH CAREGIVERS

1. Do you like your doctors?_____

2. Do you trust your doctors?_____

3. Do you think your doctors should make the final decision concerning any treatment you might need?
_____

4. How do you relate to your caregivers, including nurses, therapists, chaplains, social workers, etc.?_____
_____

5. Do you wish to make any general comments about your doctor and other health caregivers?_____

_____

C. YOUR THOUGHTS ABOUT INDEPENDENCE AND CONTROL

1. How important is independence and self-sufficiency in your life?_____

_____

2. If you were to experience decreased physical and mental abilities, how would that affect your attitude toward independence and self-sufficiency?_____

_____

3. Do you wish to make any general comments about the value of independence and control in your life?_____

_____

D. YOUR PERSONAL RELATIONSHIPS

1. Do you expect that your friends, family, and/or others will support your decisions regarding medical treatment you may need now or in the future?_____

2. Have you made any arrangements for your family or friends to make medical treatment decisions on your behalf? If so, who has agreed to make decisions for you and in what circumstances?_____

_____

3. What, if any, unfinished business from the past are you concerned about (e.g., personal and family

relationships, business and legal matters)?_____
_____

4. What role do your friends and family play in your life?
_____

5. Do you wish to make any general comments about the personal relationships in your life?_____
_____

E. YOUR OVERALL ATTITUDE TOWARD LIFE

1. What activities do you enjoy (e.g., hobbies, watching TV, etc.)?_____
_____

2. Are you happy to be alive?_____

3. Do you feel that life is worth living?_____

4. How satisfied are you with what you have achieved in your life?_____

5. What makes you laugh/cry?_____
_____

6. What do you fear most? What frightens or upsets you?
_____

7. What goals do you have for the future?_____
_____

8. Do you wish to make any general comments about your attitude toward life?_____
_____

F. YOUR ATTITUDE TOWARD ILLNESS, DYING, AND DEATH

1. What will be important to you when you are dying (e.g., physical comfort, no pain, family members present, etc.)?_____
_____

2. Where would you prefer to die?_____

3. What is your attitude toward death?_____
_____

4. How do you feel about the use of life-sustaining measures in the face of: terminal illness?_____
_____

   permanent coma?_____

   irreversible chronic illness (e.g., Alzheimer's disease)?
   _____

5. Do you wish to make any general comments about your attitude toward illness, dying, and death?_____
_____

G. YOUR RELIGIOUS BACKGROUND AND BELIEFS

1. What is your religious background?_____

2. How do your religious beliefs affect your attitude toward serious or terminal illness?_____

_____

3. Does your attitude toward death find support in your religion?_____

4. How does your faith community, church, or synagogue view the role of prayer or religious sacraments in an illness?_____

_____

5. Do you wish to make any general comments about your religious background and beliefs?_____

_____

H. YOUR LIVING ENVIRONMENT

1. What has been your living situation over the last 10 years (e.g., lived alone, lived with others, etc.)?_____

_____

2. How difficult is it for you to maintain the kind of environment for yourself that you find comfortable? Does any illness or medical problem you have now mean that it will be harder in the future?_____

_____

3. Do you wish to make any general comments about your living environment?_____

_____

I. YOUR ATTITUDE CONCERNING FINANCES

1. How much do you worry about having enough money to provide for your care?_____
_____

2. Would you prefer to spend less money on your care so that more money can be saved for the benefit of your relatives and/or friends?_____

3. Do you wish to make any general comments concerning your finances and the cost of health care?
_____

J. YOUR WISHES CONCERNING YOUR FUNERAL

1. What are your wishes concerning your funeral and burial or cremation?_____
_____

2. Have you made your funeral arrangements? If so, with whom?_____
_____

3. Do you wish to make any general comments about how you would like your funeral and burial or cremation to be arranged or conducted?_____
_____

OPTIONAL QUESTIONS

1. How would you like your obituary (announcement of your death) to read?_____

_____
_____

2. Write yourself a brief eulogy (a statement about
    yourself to be read at your funeral)._____
    _____
    _____

SUGGESTIONS FOR USE

After you have completed this form, you may wish to provide
copies to your doctors and other health caregivers, your
family, your friends, and your attorney. If you have a Living
Will or Durable Power of Attorney for Health Care Decisions,
you may wish to attach a copy of this form to those
documents.

VALUES HISTORY FORM:
SUGGESTIONS FOR USE

Here, as you requested, is the **Values History Form**
developed at the Center for Health Law and Ethics,
University of New Mexico School of Law. The form is **not a
legal document**, although it may be used to supplement a
Living Will or a Durable Power of Attorney for Health Care,
if you have these. Also, the Values History Form **is not
copyrighted,** and you are encouraged to make additional
copies for friends and relatives to use.

The Importance of Completing a Medical Directive

Thinking about and clarifying your values in an advance directive is important. Your unique ways of thinking about the world profoundly affect the decisions you make every day. But another ingredient is also important in writing an effective advance directive: considering which medical treatments you do or do not want to be used in the event you become unable to make competent medical decisions for yourself.

Dr. Linda Emanuel and Dr. Ezekiel Emanuel developed "The Medical Directive"[1] that follows to aid people in clarifying their thinking on the use of various medical treatments. It can help change the focus from your values (what is important to you) to your treatment preferences (which types of treatment you do or do not want). It can also be used as a discussion starter between you and your physician as you complete an advance directive.

Although "The Medical Directive" is copyrighted, the authors have granted me permission to reproduce it for educational awareness only. If you believe this sample medical directive would be helpful to you, copies of the form may be obtained from the Harvard Medical School Health Publication Group, P.O. Box 380, Boston, Massachusetts 02117, at 2 copies for $5 or 5 copies for $10; bulk orders are available.

The Medical Directive

Introduction

As part of a person's right to self-determination, every adult may accept or refuse any recommended medical treatment. This is relatively easy when people are well and can speak. Unfortunately, during serious illness they are often unconscious or otherwise unable to communicate their wishes—at the very time when many critical decisions need to be made.

The Medical Directive allows you to record your wishes regarding various types of medical treatment in several representative situations so that your desires can be respected. It also lets you appoint someone to make medical decisions for you if you should become unable to make them on your own.

The Medical Directive comes into effect only if you become incompetent (unable to make decisions or express your wishes), and you can change it at any time until then. As long as you are competent, you should discuss your care directly with your physician.

Completing the form

You should, if possible, complete the form in the context of a discussion with your physician. Ideally, this should occur in the presence of your proxy. This lets your physician and your proxy know how you think about these decisions, and it provides you and your physician with the opportunity to give or clarify relevant personal or medical information. You may wish to discuss the issues with your family, friends, or religious mentor.

The Medical Directive contains six illness situations that include incompetence. For each one, you consider possible interventions and goals of medical care. Situations A and B involve coma; C and D, dementia; E, chronic disability; E and F, temporary inability to make decisions.

The interventions are divided into six groups: 1) cardiopulmonary resuscitation or major surgery; 2) mechanical breathing or dialysis; 3) blood transfusions or blood products; 4) artificial nutrition and hydration; 5) simple diagnostic tests or antibiotics; and 6) pain medications, even if they dull consciousness and indirectly shorten life. Most of these treatments are described briefly. If you have further questions, consult your physician.

Your wishes for treatment options (I want this treatment; I want this treatment tried, but stopped if there is no clear improvement; I am undecided; I do not want this treatment) should be indicated. If you choose a trial of treatment, you should understand that this indicates you want the treatment *withdrawn* if your physician and proxy believe you would have agreed that it has become futile.

The Personal Statement section allows you to mention anything that you consider important to tell those who may make decisions for you concerning the limits of your life and the goals of intervention. For example, your description of insufferable disability in the Personal Statement will aid your health-care team in understanding exactly when to avoid interventions you may have declined in situation E. Or if, in situation B, you wish to define "uncertain chance" with numerical probability, you may do so here.

Next you may express your preferences concerning organ donation. Do you wish to donate your body or some or all of your organs after your death? If so, for what purpose(s) and to which physician or institution? If not, this should also be indicated in the appropriate box.

In the final section you may designate one or more proxy decision makers, who would be asked to make choices under circumstances in which your wishes are unclear. You can indicate whether the decisions of the proxy should override, or be overridden by, your wishes if there are differences. And should you name more than one proxy, you can state who is to have the final say if there is disagreement. Your proxy must understand that this role usually involves making judgments that you would have made for yourself, had you been able—and making them by the criteria you have outlined. Proxy decisions should ideally be made in discussion with your family, friends, and physician.

What to do with the form

Once you have completed the form, you and two adult witnesses (other than your proxy) who have no interest in your estate need to sign and date it.

Many states have legislation covering documents of this sort. To determine the laws in your state, you should call the office of its attorney general or consult a lawyer. If your state has a statutory document, you may wish to use the Medical Directive and append it to this form.

You should give a copy of the completed document to your physician. His or her signature is desirable but not mandatory. The Directive should be placed in your medical records and flagged so that anyone who might be involved in your care can be aware of its presence. Your proxy, a family member, and/or a friend should also have a copy. In addition, you may want to carry a wallet card noting that you have such a document and where it can be found.

MY MEDICAL DIRECTIVE

This Medical Directive expresses, and shall stand for, my wishes regarding medical treatments in the event that illness should make me unable to communicte them directly. I make this Directive, being 18 years or more of age, of sound mind, and appreciating the consequences of my decisions.

1. **Cardiopulmonary resuscitation** (chest compressions, drugs, electric shocks, and artificial breathing aimed at reviving a person who is on the point of dying), **or major surgery** (for example, removing the gall bladder or part of the colon)

2. **Mechanical breathing** (respiration by machine, through a tube in the throat), or dialysis (cleaning the blood by machine or by fluid passed through the belly)

3. **Blood tranfusions of blood products**

4. **Artificial nutrition and hydration** (given through a tube in a vein or in the stomach)

5. **Simple diagnostic test** (for example, blood test or x-rays), **or antibiotics** (drugs to fight infection)

6. **Pain medications, even if they dull consciousness and indirectly shorten my life**

THE GOAL OF MEDICAL CARE SHOULD BE (*check one*):

SITUATION A

If I am in a coma, a persistent vegetative state and, in the opinion of my physician and two consultants, have no known hope of regaining awareness and higher mental functions no matter what is done, then my wishes — for this and any additional illness would be:

I want	I want treatment tried. If no clear improvement, stop.	I am undecided	I do not want
	Not applicable		
	Not applicable		
	Not applicable		
	Not applicable		

___ Prolong life; treat everything
___ choose quality of life over longevity
___ provide comfort care only
___ other (please specify):

MY MEDICAL DIRECTIVE

This Medical Directive expresses, and shall stand for, my wishes regarding medical treatments in the event that illness should make me unable to communicte them directly. I make this Directive, being 18 years or more of age, of sound mind, and appreciating the consequences of my decisions.

1. **Cardiopulmonary resuscitation** (chest compressions, drugs, electric shocks, and artificial breathing aimed at reviving a person who is on the point of dying), **or major surgery** (for example, removing the gall bladder or part of the colon)

2. **Mechanical breathing** (respiration by machine, through a tube in the throat), or dialysis (cleaning the blood by machine or by fluid passed through the belly)

3. **Blood tranfusions of blood products**

4. **Artificial nutrition and hydration** (given through a tube in a vein or in the stomach)

5. **Simple diagnostic test** (for example, blood test or x-rays), **or antibiotics** (drugs to fight infection)

6. **Pain medications, even if they dull consciousness and indirectly shorten my life**

THE GOAL OF MEDICAL CARE SHOULD BE (*check one*):

SITUATION B

If I am in a coma and, in the opinion of my physician and two consultants, have a slight, but uncertain chance of regaining some higher mental functions, a somewhat greater chance of surviving with permanent brain damage, and a much greater chance of not recovering at all, then my wishes — if medically reasonable — for this and any additional illness would be:

I want	I want treatment tried. If no clear improvement, stop.	I am undecided	I do not want
	Not applicable		
	Not applicable		
	Not applicable		
	Not applicable		

____ Prolong life; treat everything
____ choose quality of life over longevity
____ provide comfort care only
____ other (please specify):

_____

1. **Cardiopulmonary resuscitation** (chest compressions, drugs, electric shocks, and artificial breathing aimed at reviving a person who is on the point of dying), **or major surgery** (for example, removing the gall bladder or part of the colon)

2. **Mechanical breathing** (respiration by machine, through a tube in the throat), or dialysis (cleaning the blood by machine or by fluid passed through the belly)

3. **Blood tranfusions of blood products**

4. **Artificial nutrition and hydration** (given through a tube in a vein or in the stomach)

5. **Simple diagnostic test** (for example, blood test or x-rays), **or antibiotics** (drugs to fight infection)

6. **Pain medications, even if they dull consciousness and indirectly shorten my life**

THE GOAL OF MEDICAL CARE
SHOULD BE (*check one*):

SITUATION C

If I have brain damage or some brain disease that in the opinion of my physician and two consultants cannot be reversed and that makes me unable to recognize people, to speak meaningfully to them, or to live independently, *and I also have a terminal illness,* then my wishes — if medically reasonable — for this and any additional illness would be:

I want	I want treatment tried. If no clear improvement, stop.	I am undecided	I do not want
	Not applicable		
	Not applicable		
	Not applicable		
	Not applicable		

____ Prolong life; treat everything
____ choose quality of life over longevity
____ provide comfort care only
____ other (please specify):

_____

MY MEDICAL DIRECTIVE

This Medical Directive expresses, and shall stand for, my wishes regarding medical treatments in the event that illness should make me unable to communicte them directly. I make this Directive, being 18 years or more of age, of sound mind, and appreciating the consequences of my decisions.

1. **Cardiopulmonary resuscitation** (chest compressions, drugs, electric shocks, and artificial breathing aimed at reviving a person who is on the point of dying), **or major surgery** (for example, removing the gall bladder or part of the colon)

2. **Mechanical breathing** (respiration by machine, through a tube in the throat), or dialysis (cleaning the blood by machine or by fluid passed through the belly)

3. **Blood tranfusions of blood products**

4. **Artificial nutrition and hydration** (given through a tube in a vein or in the stomach)

5. **Simple diagnostic test** (for example, blood test or x-rays), **or antibiotics** (drugs to fight infection)

6. **Pain medications, even if they dull consciousness and indirectly shorten my life**

THE GOAL OF MEDICAL CARE SHOULD BE (*check one*):

SITUATION D

If I have brain damage or some brain disease that in the opinion of my physician and two consultants cannot be reversed and that makes me unable to recognize people, to speak meaningfully to them, or to live independently, *and I have no terminal illness*, then my wishes — if medically reasonable — for this and any additional illness would be:

I want	I want treatment tried. If no clear improvement, stop.	I am undecided	I do not want
	Not applicable		
	Not applicable		
	Not applicable		
	Not applicable		

___ Prolong life; treat everything
___ choose quality of life over longevity
___ provide comfort care only
___ other (please specify):

_____

MY MEDICAL DIRECTIVE

This Medical Directive expresses, and shall stand for, my wishes regarding medical treatments in the event that illness should make me unable to communicte them directly. I make this Directive, being 18 years or more of age, of sound mind, and appreciating the consequences of my decisions.

1. **Cardiopulmonary resuscitation** (chest compressions, drugs, electric shocks, and artificial breathing aimed at reviving a person who is on the point of dying), **or major surgery** (for example, removing the gall bladder or part of the colon)

2. **Mechanical breathing** (respiration by machine, through a tube in the throat), or dialysis (cleaning the blood by machine or by fluid passed through the belly)

3. **Blood tranfusions of blood products**

4. **Artificial nutrition and hydration** (given through a tube in a vein or in the stomach)

5. **Simple diagnostic test** (for example, blood test or x-rays), **or antibiotics** (drugs to fight infection)

6. **Pain medications, even if they dull consciousness and indirectly shorten my life**

THE GOAL OF MEDICAL CARE SHOULD BE (*check one*):

SITUATION E

If, in the opinion of my physician and two consultants, I have an incurable chronic illness that involves mental disability or physical suffering and ultimately causes death, and in addition I have an illness that is immediately life threatening but reversible, and I am temporarily unable to make decisions, then my wishes — if medically reasonable — would be:

I want	I want treatment tried. If no clear improvement, stop.	I am undecided	I do not want
	Not applicable		
	Not applicable		
	Not applicable		
	Not applicable		

____ Prolong life; treat everything
____ choose quality of life over longevity
____ provide comfort care only
____ other (please specify):

_____

MY MEDICAL DIRECTIVE

This Medical Directive expresses, and shall stand for, my wishes regarding medical treatments in the event that illness should make me unable to communicte them directly. I make this Directive, being 18 years or more of age, of sound mind, and appreciating the consequences of my decisions.

1. **Cardiopulmonary resuscitation** (chest compressions, drugs, electric shocks, and artificial breathing aimed at reviving a person who is on the point of dying), **or major surgery** (for example, removing the gall bladder or part of the colon)

2. **Mechanical breathing** (respiration by machine, through a tube in the throat), or dialysis (cleaning the blood by machine or by fluid passed through the belly)

3. **Blood tranfusions of blood products**

4. **Artificial nutrition and hydration** (given through a tube in a vein or in the stomach)

5. **Simple diagnostic test** (for example, blood test or x-rays), **or antibiotics** (drugs to fight infection)

6. **Pain medications, even if they dull consciousness and indirectly shorten my life**

THE GOAL OF MEDICAL CARE SHOULD BE (*check one*):

SITUATION F

If I am in my current state of health (*describe briefly*)_____
_____ and then have an illness that,
in the opinion of my physician and two consultants, is life
threatening but reversible, and I am temporarily unable to
make decisions, then my wishes — if medically reasonable
— would be:

I want	I want treatment tried. If no clear improvement, stop.	I am undecided	I do not want
	Not applicable		
	Not applicable		
	Not applicable		
	Not applicable		

____ Prolong life; treat everything
____ choose quality of life over longevity
____ provide comfort care only
____ other (please specify):

_____

MY PERSONAL STATEMENT
(use another page if necessary)

Please mention anything that would be important for your physician and your proxy to know. In particular, try to answer the following questions: 1) What medical conditions, if any, would make living so unpleasant that you would want life-sustaining treatment *withheld?* (Intractable pain? Irreversible mental damage? Inability to share love? Dependence on others? Another condition you would regard as intolerable?) 2) Under what medical circumstances would you want to *stop* interventions that might already have been started?

_____

_____

_____

_____

Should there be any difference between my preferences detailed in the illness situations and those understood from my goals or from my personal statement, I wish my treatment selections/my goals/my personal statement *(please delete as appropriate)* to be given greater weight.

When I am dying, I would like—if my proxy and my health care team think it is reasonable—to be cared for:

☐ at home or in a hospice
☐ in a nursing home
☐ in a hospital
☐ other *(please specify)*:_____

ORGAN DONATION
(please check boxes and fill in blanks where appropriate)

I hereby make this anatomical gift, to take effect after my death:

I give   ☐ my body
           ☐ any needed organs or parts
           ☐ the following parts:_____

to   ☐ the following person or institution:_____
           _____

           ☐ the physician in attendance at my death
           ☐ the hospital in which I die
           ☐ the following physician, hospital storage
              bank, or other medical institution:_____
           _____

for   ☐ any purpose authorized by law
           ☐ therapy of another person
           ☐ medical education
           ☐ transplantation
           ☐ research

____ I do not wish to make any anatomical gift from my body.

DURABLE POWER OF ATTORNEY FOR HEALTH CARE

I appoint as my proxy decision maker(s):

_____

Name and Address

and (*optional*)

_____

Name and Address

I direct my proxy to make health-care decisions based on his/her assessment of my personal wishes. If my personal desires are unknown, my proxy is to make health-care decisions for me based on his/her best guess as to my wishes. My proxy shall have the authority to make all health-care decisions for me, including decisions about life-sustaining treatment, if I am unable to make them myself. My proxy's authority becomes effective if my attending physician determines in writing that I lack the capacity to make or communicate health-care decisions. My proxy is then to have the same authority to make health-care decisions as I would if I had the capacity to make them, EXCEPT *(list the limitations, if any, you wish to place on your proxy's authority)*:

Should there be any disagreement between the wishes I have indicated in this document and the decisions favored by my above-named proxy, I wish my proxy to have authority over my written statements / I wish my written statements to bind my proxy. *(Please delete as necessary.)* If I have appointed more than one proxy and there is disagreement between

their wishes, _____ shall have final
authority.

Signed:

_____

Signature   Printed Name

_____

Address   Date

Witness:

_____

Signature   Printed Name

_____

Address   Date

Witness:

_____

Signature   Printed Name

_____

Address   Date

Physician *(optional)*

I am _____'s physician. I have seen this advance care document and have had an opportunity to discuss his/her preferences regarding medical interventions at the end of life. If _____ _____ becomes incompetent, I understand that it is my duty to interpret and implement the preferences contained in this document in order to fulfill his/her wishes.

_____

Signature   Printed Name

_____

Address   Date

CHAPTER 8

Types of Advance Directives

Once you have thought about your personal values and medical treatment preferences, it will be easy for you to translate them into an effective communication tool—the advance directive of your choice—that you can share with health care professionals.

Advance directives currently come in three forms: Durable Power of Attorney for Health Care/Proxy Directive (DPAHC); Combination Durable Power of Attorney for Health Care/Instructive Directive; and the Living Will/Instructive Directive. In this chapter we will explore each type of advance directive and include sample forms of each. *Please note: these model forms are to assist you in understanding the issues. They in no way render legal advice, because laws regarding advance directives vary somewhat from state to state. Therefore, the forms are included without warranty of any kind. You will need to research the legal requirements of advance directives in your state before writing the directive you believe is best for you. In no event shall the author or publisher be liable or responsible for any problems that arise from your use of the following sample forms.*

The following sample advance directives are important legal documents. If completed properly according to the laws of the state in which you reside, each directive will remain valid indefinitely or until such time as it is revoked by you. (Note: If you reside in more than one state, you may need a separate advance directive to meet the legal requirements of each.) So you should know these facts:

1. Both the Durable Power of Attorney for Health Care/Proxy Directive and the Combination Durable Power of Attorney for Health Care/Instructive Directive give the person that you (the principal) designate as your agent (surrogate, proxy, attorney-in-fact) the power to make health care decisions for you. Your agent must act consistently with your desires as stated in this document. There may be restrictions on who can be appointed to be your surrogate. For example, generally no health care professional providing for your care can become your surrogate unless he or she is your legal spouse.

2. Subject to your stated desires, the Durable Power of Attorney for Health Care/Proxy Directive and the Combination Durable Power of Attorney for Health Care/Instructive Directive give your agent the power to consent to a physician's recommendation to withhold treatment or to stop treatment necessary to keep you alive.

3. You have the right to make medical and other health care decisions for yourself as long as you can give informed consent with respect to the particular decision. No treatment may be given to you over your objection.

4. A court may take away the power of your agent to

make health care decisions for you if your agent: authorizes something that is illegal; acts contrary to your known desires; or, where your desires are not known, does anything that is clearly contrary to your best interests.

5. You have the right to revoke the authority of your agent at any time. The directive will remain valid indefinitely or until such time as it is revoked by you.

6. If you are a patient in a skilled nursing facility, you may need to secure the signature of a patient advocate or ombudsman.

7. If you are a conservatee and want to select your conservator as your agent or alternate agent, you must obtain an attorney's certification.

8. Generally speaking, a witness should not be a health care professional.

Durable Power of Attorney for Health Care/Proxy Directive

The concept of designating one person to assume legal responsibility for an aspect of another person's business dealings has a long history in the United States. A Durable Power of Attorney for Financial Affairs allows a competent person to transfer his or her authority to make financial decisions to another individual (proxy) in the event the person executing the document becomes noncompetent or incapacitated. Every state currently has laws that allow people to designate a proxy for financial matters.

The Durable Power of Attorney for Health Care/Proxy Directive seeks to perform a similar function. This type of advance directive allows the person executing it (the "principal") to legally designate a specific person known synony-mously as an "agent," "surrogate," "proxy," or "attorney-in-fact" who will carry out the principal's health care decisions should the principal become unable to make informed choices. This document usually grants full authority to the designated surrogate or attorney-in-fact to make all health care decisions, subject to any limitations the principal states in the document. No court, as of this writing, has ever invalidated a durable power of attorney that was specifically designed to appoint a surrogate for health care decisions.

The Durable Power of Attorney for Health Care/Proxy Directive has advantages over a solely instructional directive such as a Living Will because it gives the surrogate the same decision-making authority that the patient would have had if the patient were able to make informed choices. This type of document, therefore, gives the surrogate legal authority to agree to or to refuse treatment on behalf of a patient who lacks decision-making capacity, subject to any stated limits. Because health care professionals are able to talk with a patient's designated, legal representative who is empowered to analyze information and make decisions, there is no second-guessing of instructions that may not fit the patient's exact clinical situation.

The Durable Power of Attorney for Health Care/Proxy Directive that grants blanket authority to the agent or sur-rogate is easy to implement; when the principal is deemed unable to make competent medical decisions, the surrogate takes over and makes all medical decisions. This type of advance directive also protects health care professionals who follow a surrogate's directions concerning life-sustaining treatment. Naming a particular person to be the designated surrogate decision maker also prevents problems if family members disagree on a course of treatment. The principal may not want to choose his or her spouse or adult child as the surrogate if this could create an undue emotional burden for the family member. A good friend may be the best choice.

It would be prudent for the principal to designate both a primary surrogate and an alternate in the event the primary surrogate could not fulfill his or her obligation. Also, any person writing a Durable Power of Attorney for Health Care/Proxy Directive should speak at length with the person he or she chooses as a surrogate (or agent) so that the surrogate will be familiar with the principal's treatment preferences and personal values. (Following is a sample completed form and a blank form for you to complete is in Appendix A.)

DURABLE POWER OF ATTORNEY FOR HEALTH CARE/PROXY DIRECTIVE

I, [Full Name] _John David Doe_ , residing at Address _123 East St._
City _Anytown_ State _CA_ Zip _12345_ , appoint as my Agent (attorney-in-fact): [Agent's Full Name] _James Robert Brown_ , of [His/Her Address] _456 West St._ .
City _Anytown_ State _CA_ Zip _12345_
Telephone Number _(123) 456-7890_

If my Agent is unwilling or unable to serve, then I appoint as my alternate Agent (attorney-in-fact): [Alternate Agent's Full Name] _Mary Ann Smith_ ,of [Address] _789 North St._ .
City _Anytown_ State _CA_ Zip _12345_ .
Telephone Number _(123) 876-5432_

My Agent shall have the authority to make health care decisions for me, subject to any limitations I state below, if I am unable to make decisions for myself. My Agent's authority becomes effective if it is confirmed in writing, by two physicians, that I lack the capacity to make or to communicate informed health care decisions. My Agent is then to have the same authority to make health care decisions as I would if I had the capacity to make them, except: [here list the limitations, if any, you wish to place on your Agent's authority]: __None__

_____.

I direct my Agent to make decisions based upon my Agent's understanding of my personal values. If my personal values are unknown, my Agent is to make decisions on the basis of his/her assessment of my best interests. Photocopies of this Durable Power of Attorney for Health Care/Proxy Instructive shall have the same force and effect as the original.

Signed [Your Name]___*John David Doe*___

Date ___*31 February 1997*___

WITNESS STATEMENT

We, the undersigned, declare under the penalty of perjury that the Declarant who signed this advance directive did so in our presence, and that the Declarant appears to be of sound mind and under no constraints or undue influence. We did not sign the Declarant's signature for or at the direction of the Declarant. We are at least eighteen (18) years of age and are not related to the Declarant by blood or marriage, entitled to any portion of the estate of the Declarant under any will of the Declarant or codicil thereto now existing or by operation of law, or directly financially responsible for the Declarant's medical care. We are not the Declarant's attending physician, an employee of the attending physician, or an employee of the health facility in which the Declarant is a patient. Neither of us is named as the Agent or Alternate Agent in this document.

In our presence this _31_ day of _February_, 19_97_.

I sign my name to this advance directive for health care on this _31_ day of _February_, 19_97_.

WITNESS 1

Name [Print] _Sue Jones_

Signature _Sue Jones_

Address _109 South St._

City _Anytown_ State _CA_ Zip _12345_

Telephone Number _(123) 654 - 3210_

WITNESS 2

Name [Print] _Joe Johnson_

Signature _Joe Johnson_

Address _876 First St._

City _Anytown_ State _CA_ Zip _12345_

Telephone Number _(123) 543 - 2100_

Use the following if your state requires that this document be acknowledged before a Notary Public:

Before me, _Jane Taylor_, on this
[insert name of Notary Public]

_31_ day of _February_ 19_97_, personally appeared _John Doe_,[name of Declarant completing this form] known to me to be the

108

Declarant whose name is signed to the foregoing instrument, and who, in my presence, did subscribe his/her name to the attached Durable Power of Attorney for Health Care/Proxy Directive on this date, and that said Declarant at the time of execution of said Declaration was over the age of eighteen (18) years and of sound mind.

Seal   Notary Public

PHYSICIAN STATEMENT

I, the undersigned, am the physician of __John Doe__
_____. I have seen this document and discussed it with __John Doe_____.
If __John Doe_____ becomes unable to make competent decisions, I understand that it is my duty to be guided by this advance directive.
Signature__Marv Mmn   MD_____

Combination Durable Power of Attorney for Health Care/Instructive Directive

The second type of advance directive seeks to combine the "agent" designation of the Durable Power of Attorney for Health Care/Proxy Directive with the instructive material provided in the Living Will/Instructive Directive we'll look at next. In the first part of a Combination Durable Power of Attorney for Health Care/Instructive Directive, the principal designates and appoints an agent (surrogate, proxy, or attorney-in-fact) as well as an alternate agent to make competent treatment decisions if the principal should become unable to do so.

In the second section of the document, which is similar to a Living Will/Instructive Directive, the principal outlines his or her wishes, values, and treatment preferences in general terminology. The agent is to be guided by the instructive portion of the document in making decisions on behalf of the principal.

The only potential drawback of the combination type of advance directive is that it is difficult to document desires concerning every possible medical treatment available. Because it is very difficult to accurately predict exact future clinical circumstances, it is advantageous for the principal to write a general statement of values in the instruction section of this type of advance directive. These values might refer to the relief of pain, a certain quality of life that the principal feels is important, and so on. Or, the principal can attach his or her completed Values History and/or Medical Directive to the Combination Durable Power of Attorney for Health Care/Instructive Directive.

One example of a general statement of treatment preference is "If I become incapacitated to the point that I am in a persistent vegetative state with no possibility of regaining any conscious awareness, I do not want to be kept alive with a feeding tube which artificially supplies nutrition and hydration." By stating this clearly, the principal can be sure that his or her wishes will be carried out if he or she can no longer make competent medical treatment decisions. Other examples of general statements might be "I do not want life-sustaining treatment to be provided if the burdens outweigh the benefits" or "I do not desire futile treatment." It's important for the principal to be specific about his or her feelings concerning artificial nutrition and hydration.

An advance directive which contains an instructive element gives the principal the opportunity to state other personal preferences, too. For example, a statement giving the agent the authority to oversee the disposition of the principal's remains could be included. A statement could also be included regarding personal preferences concerning autopsy, body donation, or organ donation. (A person may wish to donate only particular organs or none at all. Some people feel comfortable leaving their bodies to a particular physician or medical institution for the purposes of medical research.) Many people will also want to be sensitive to the teachings of their religious traditions concerning burial. These preferences, clearly some of the most personal of all choices, should be discussed at length with family, friends, and the agent to ensure that one's written wishes will be followed. These are the issues and concerns dealt with at length in the Values History and Medical Directive documents found in the previous chapter. (See the following sample form in the appendix.)

111

COMBINATION DURABLE POWER OF ATTORNEY FOR HEALTH CARE/INSTRUCTIVE DIRECTIVE

I, [Your Name] __John David Doe__, a citizen of the State of __California__, residing at [Address] __123 East St.__, City __Anytown__ State __CA__ Zip __12345__, Telephone Number __(123) 246-7593__ do hereby designate and appoint as my Agent:

Name __James Robert Brown__

Address __456 West St.__

City __Anytown__ State __CA__ Zip __12345__

Telephone Number __(123) 456-7890__

This person is empowered to make health care decisions for me as authorized in this document. If my Agent is unwilling or unable to serve, then I appoint:

Name __Mary Ann Smith__

Address __789 North St.__

City __Anytown__ State __CA__ Zip __12345__

Telephone Number __(123) 876-5432__

as my Alternate Agent, empowered to make health care decisions for me as authorized in this document.

If I become unable to make informed choices concerning my health care, I hereby grant my Agent full power and authority to make health care decisions for me, subject to my preferences and values stated below.

My Agent's authority becomes effective if it is confirmed in writing, by two physicians, that I am unable to make informed choices regarding my health care.

I hereby direct my Agent to make decisions on the basis of his/her understanding of my preferences and values. My Agent should seek to weigh the burdens and benefits of any form of medical treatment and authorize those treatments that provide an overall net gain (where benefits are greater than burdens), and are in my overall best interest. Photocopies of this advance directive shall have the same force and effect as the original.

Statement of Treatment Preferences, Values, and Limitations:

(If you wish, simply attach your completed Values History/Medical Directive.) __attached__

_____

_____

(Attach additional pages if more space is needed.)

I sign my name to this advance directive for health care on this _31_ day of _February_, 19_97_.
Signature of principal: _John David Doe_

This directive will not be valid unless it is signed by two qualified adult witnesses or acknowledged by a Notary Public.

WITNESS STATEMENT

We, the undersigned, declare under the penalty of perjury that the Declarant who signed this advance directive did so in our presence, and that the Declarant appears to be of sound mind and under no constraints or undue influence. We did not sign the Declarant's signature for or at the direction of the Declarant. We are at least eighteen (18) years of age and are not related to the Declarant by blood or marriage, entitled to any portion of the estate of the Declarant under any will of the Declarant or codicil thereto now existing or by operation of law, or directly financially responsible for the Declarant's medical care. We are not the Declarant's attending physician, an employee of the attending physician, or an employee of the health facility in which the Declarant is a patient. Neither of us is named as the Agent or Alternate Agent in this document.

WITNESS 1

Name __Sue Jones_____

Address __109 South St._____

City_Anytown_____ State _CA____ Zip _12345_

Telephone Number _(123) 654·3210_____

Date __31 February 1997_____

Signature __Sue Jones_____

WITNESS 2

Name _Joe Johnson_

Address _876 First St._

City _Anytown_ State _CA_ Zip _12345_

Telephone Number _(123) 543-2100_

Date _31 February 1997_

Signature _Joe Johnson_

Signature of patient advocate or ombudsman (if needed):

Pat Williams

Date _31 February 1997_

CERTIFICATION OF ACKNOWLEDGMENT OF NOTARY PUBLIC

Use the following if your state requires that this document be acknowledged before a Notary Public:

Before me, _Jane Taylor_, on this
[insert name of Notary Public]

_31_ day of _February_, 19_97_, personally appeared
John Doe , [name of
Declarant completing this form] known to me to be the
Declarant whose name is signed to the foregoing instrument,
and who, in my presence, did subscribe his/her name to the
attached Combination Durable Power of Attorney for Health

Care/Instructive Directive on this date, and that said Declarant at the time of execution of said Declaration was over the age of eighteen (18) years and of sound mind.

Seal   Notary Public

PHYSICIAN STATEMENT

I, the undersigned, am the physician of _John Doe_.
John Doe. I have seen this document and discussed it with _John Doe_.
If _John Doe_ becomes unable to make competent decisions, I understand that it is my duty to be guided by this advance directive.
Signature _Mm Mw MD_

The Living Will/Instructive Directive

In this type of instructive directive, a competent adult declares what types of life-sustaining treatments he or she does or does not want to receive in the event he or she is unable to make informed medical treatment decisions sometime in the future. This document usually pertains to a terminal, incurable illness.

Nothing is more important in this variety of advance directive than a clear, concise declaration of a person's treatment preferences. Conversely, this is also one of the shortcomings of this type of advance directive. A person completing a Living Will must accurately predict the medical interventions that might be available to postpone his or her death. Often a Living Will is worded so generally that it's difficult to apply to an actual medical situation where a specific treatment is being considered.

One possible way a person can avoid this type of ambiguity is to state his or her values in broader terms that may apply to a variety of situations. For instance, a possible statement might be "I do not want life-sustaining treatment to be provided if the burdens outweigh the benefits. I want my care givers to consider the relief of my suffering and the quality of my life in making decisions concerning my treatment."

Although the Living Will form of advance directive encourages people to document their values, virtually all Living Wills suffer from major shortcomings:

In some states, they are only applicable to those who are "terminally ill."

Some states require specific documentation to limit the provision for artificial nutrition and hydration.

A Living Will makes no provision for the person creating

it to designate a surrogate to make treatment decisions on his or her behalf.

In the light of these shortcomings, it is accurate to say that the Living Will type of advance directive is simply a statement of a person's treatment preferences and may or may not accurately reflect his or her future situation. Living Wills were the first type of advance directive available. They were a good start, but the current medical, legal, and ethical consensus indicates that a different type of advance directive, such as a Combination Durable Power of Attorney for Health Care/Instructive Directive, will communicate treatment desires more effectively.

THE LIVING WILL/INSTRUCTIVE DIRECTIVE

Declaration made this _31_ day of _February_ , 19_97_.

I, _John David Doe_ , being of sound mind, willfully and voluntarily make known my desires that my dying shall not be artificially prolonged under circumstances set forth below, and do declare:

If I should have an incurable and irreversible condition that has been diagnosed by two physicians and that will result in my death within a relatively short time without the administration of life-sustaining treatment or that has produced an irreversible coma or persistent vegetative state, and I am no longer able to make competent decisions regarding my medical treatment, I direct my physician to withhold or withdraw treatment that only prolongs the process of dying or the irreversible coma or persistent vegetative state I am in and that is not necessary for my comfort or to alleviate pain.

If I should have an incurable or irreversible condition or should be in an irreversible coma or persistent vegetative state, I direct my attending physician to withhold or withdraw artificially administered nutrition and hydration that only prolongs the process of dying.

_____John David Doe_____ (Sign here to indicate you would not want tube feeding—artificial nutrition and hydration.)

Declarant's statement of values and treatment preferences

List here any of your treatment preferences or values concerning quality of life, or attach your completed Values History and/or Medical Directive.

attached
_____
_____

In the absence of my ability to give directions regarding the use of such life-sustaining procedures, it is my intention that this declaration shall be honored by my family and physicians as the final expression of my legal right to refuse medical treatment and to accept the consequences of such refusal.

I understand the full import of this declaration, and I am emotionally and mentally competent to make this declaration.

Signed _John David Doe_

Address _123 East St._

City _Anytown_ State _CA_ Zip _12345_

Telephone Number _(123) 246-8101_

WITNESS STATEMENT

We, the undersigned, declare under the penalty of perjury that the Declarant who signed this advance directive did so in our presence, and that the Declarant appears to be of sound mind and under no constraints or undue influence.

We did not sign the Declarant's signature for or at the direction of the Declarant. We are at least eighteen (18) years of age and are not related to the Declarant by blood or marriage, entitled to any portion of the estate of the Declarant under any will of the Declarant or codicil thereto now existing or by operation of law, or directly financially responsible for the Declarant's medical care. We are not the Declarant's attending physician, an employee of the attending physician, or an employee of the health facility in which the Declarant is a patient. Neither of us is named as the Agent or Alternate Agent in this document.

Witness (please print) _Sue Jones_

Signature _Sue Jones_

Address _109 South St._

City _Anytown_ State _CA_ Zip _12345_

Telephone Number _(123) 654 - 3210_

Witness (please print) _Joe Johnson_

Signature _Joe Johnson_

Address _876 First St._

City _Anytown_ State _CA_ Zip _12345_

Telephone Number _(123) 543·2100_

Use the following if your state requires that this document be acknowledged before a Notary Public:

Before me, ____*Jane   Taylor*_____, on this

[insert name of Notary Public]

_31_ day of _*February*___ , 19_97_, personally appeared,
____*John   David   Doe*_____

[name of Declarant completing this form] known to me to be the Declarant whose name is signed to the foregoing instrument, and who, in my presence, did subscribe his/her name to the attached Living Will on this date, and that said Declarant at the time of execution of said Declaration was over the age of eighteen (18) years and of sound mind.

Seal   Notary Public

PHYSICIAN STATEMENT

I, the undersigned, am the physician of _*John   Doe*___
_____. I have seen this document and discussed it with_*John   Doe*_____.
If _*John   Doe*_____ becomes unable to make competent decisions, I understand that it is my duty to be guided by this advance directive.
Signature_____

CHAPTER 9

Christian Belief and Treatment Decisions

At this time, there is a need for a new emphasis on the role of theology in decisions concerning bioethical issues. Religious beliefs have always played an important role in the history of humankind, often forming the foundational principles that enable people to live together in community. As we have seen, Christian theology has made a necessary contribution to the present consensus regarding life-sustaining treatment.

However, this theological influence is now waning, due in part to the authority and influence given to court decisions in the area of bioethics. Daniel Callahan, director of The Hastings Center, sees the recent disappearance of religion in public discourse as a triple threat. He believes this absence of religious perspective leaves us too heavily dependent on law as the working source of morality. It also leaves us without the accumulated wisdom and knowledge that are the fruit of long-established religious traditions. Finally, it forces us to pretend that we are not members of communities with particular moral values. We all have moral "roots"—often based on religion. In fact, they form the foundation of our democracy.[1]

As we've seen, Christian theology has a long tradition of considering moral problems such as the meaning of suffering, sickness, and death within the context of humankind's relationship with God. These understandings of moral problems can make a significant contribution to the current discussions of bioethical issues. Theological insights go beyond the basic principles of bioethics. In fact, most ethical principles develop from a corresponding theological concept concerning the way in which God interacts with the world.

For instance, the patient's right to self-determination, or the principle of autonomy, is one of the grounding principles in the discussion of treatment options, as is evident in the emerging consensus and recent legislation. The principle of self-determination or autonomy is closely related to the theological concept that all of humankind is created in the image of God. Let's take a closer look at the concept of the image of God and how it relates to bioethical discussion.

The concept first appears in Genesis 1:26–27: "Then God said, 'Let us make humankind in our image, according to our likeness. . . .' So God created humankind in his image, in the image of God he created them; male and female he created them." The theological concept of the image of God contains a rich web of meaning that goes beyond merely stating that all people have the right to make personal choices. The following, an excerpt from a special supplement entitled "Theology, Religious Traditions, and Bioethics" released by The Hastings Center, comments on how this biblical tradition relates to the ethical principle of autonomy:

> Central convictions of theological anthropology in biblical traditions, such as that human beings are created in the image of God, support the notion of intrinsic human dignity and respect for personal choice conveyed in bioethics discourse by the principle of autonomy.[2]

For people of faith, this means that every person reflects the essence of God, which is love. Whereas the principle of autonomy is primarily rational, the concept of the image of God is relational.

God chooses to create people who have the capacity for relationship with one another and with God. God creates humankind in such a way that people are empowered to be co-creators with God. By possessing a portion of God's essence, people are capable of making choices that are nurturing and redeeming—choices that reflect the image of God. People may not always exercise their freedom in responsible ways, but they have the freedom to decide, which is a very important part of being created in God's image. God creates people to be free moral agents, not puppets.

The biblical concept of justice, which can expand our thinking on ethical principles, includes God's preferential option for the poor and those devalued by society. Biblical justice means going beyond societal norms in showing care to sick people. Biblical justice entails witnessing to the love of God through concrete acts of mercy. The prophet Jeremiah offers these words of warning to those who would hide in God's temple while treating their neighbors with apathy or injustice:

> For if you truly amend your ways and your doings, if you truly act justly one with another, if you do not oppress the alien, the orphan, and the widow, or shed innocent blood in this place, and if you do not go after other gods to your own hurt, then I will dwell with you in this place, in the land that I gave of old to your ancestors forever and ever. (Jer. 7:5–7)

Jesus rephrased Jeremiah's advice when addressing a lawyer's question:

> Just then a lawyer stood up to test Jesus. "Teacher," he said, "what must I do to inherit eternal life?" He said to him, "What is written in the law? What do you read there?" He answered, "You shall love the Lord your God with all your heart, and with all your soul, and with all your strength, and with all your mind; and your neighbor as yourself." And he said to him, "You have given the right answer; do this, and you will live." (Luke 10:25–28)

Although the ethical principle of beneficence conveys an obligation to do no harm to the patient and to care for the welfare of others, the biblical concept of justice goes beyond the ethical principle and establishes the standard of love for one's neighbor. The biblical tradition makes it clear that in order for us to live in community, we must have a level of concern that goes beyond superficial gestures and legal standards of justice. Biblical justice and the love of our neighbor demand that we think of creative ways to care for seriously ill individuals who are suffering.

This means that we should think of ways to physically and emotionally comfort those who suffer from serious illness. Whereas the ethical principle of beneficence establishes a minimum level of caring for others, the biblical concept of justice and love obligates us to assume personal sacrifice, to risk, and to make every possible effort to reflect God's love. Jesus reflected God's love in this way to all people, thus becoming the model for all who would seek fellowship with God.

Almost all of the religious traditions in our society have at their core a fundamental commitment to love God and neighbor. I see this as the most important contribution of theology to bioethics. Theology can impress upon us the importance of caring, of supporting one another through the experiences of suffering and death. It is only through actively loving one another in "the darkest valley," mentioned in Psalm 23:4, that we fulfill our purpose for being alive. Theology can contribute profound insights about the ultimate meaning of life, even in the midst of suffering and death.

For people of faith, the theological concepts of self-determination, justice, and love can form a framework for understanding the complex issues and personal dynamics that surround any bioethical dilemma. I advocate a framework that rests on two main points: compassion and common sense.

Compassion

My understanding of the gospel of Jesus Christ has at its center the fact that Jesus was a channel for the love of God and that He demonstrated that love in all He did through concrete acts of compassion.

The English word compassion comes from two Latin words, com ("with") and pati ("to suffer"). The word clearly means "to suffer with," or specifically, "to suffer with another person." To have compassion means to share in the person's affliction, to bring comfort. Webster's New Collegiate Dictionary defines the word this way: "Sympathetic consciousness of others' distress together with a desire to alleviate it, the deep feeling of sharing the suffering of another."3

The law of Christ is the law of love that seeks to treat people with respect and caring comfort, especially those who are seriously ill. To be present with people who are seriously ill and dying is not easy, but it is what the followers of Jesus Christ are called to do. As Paul writes in Galatians 6:2, "Bear one another's burdens, and in this way you will fulfill the law of Christ."

One of the most well-documented aspects of Jesus' ministry was His healing ministry. The Synoptic Gospels contain thirteen narratives of how Jesus healed "fever, leprosy, paralysis, withered hand, bent back, hemorrhage, deafness and dumbness, dropsy, severed ear, and a sickness near death or paralysis."[4] Jesus used different methods to carry out His ministry of compassion. Sometimes He healed by word. He said to the man with the withered hand, "Stretch out your hand," and the hand was restored (Mark 3:5). When a leper came to Him, Jesus was "moved with pity" and touched him, and immediately the leprosy left him (Mark 1:40–42). Sometimes Jesus used physical means in addition to touching, as in the case of the deaf man. Jesus "put his fingers into his ears, and he spat and touched his tongue. Then looking up to heaven, he sighed and said to him, 'Ephphatha,' that is, 'Be opened.' And immediately his ears were opened, his tongue was released, and he spoke plainly" (Mark 7:33–35).

Despite His different methods, there is one consistent aspect to Jesus' healings: They were the result of "power." The word most often used to describe the mighty deeds of Jesus in the Synoptic Gospels is the Greek word *dunamis*, which means "power." The Gospel writers and Jesus Himself understood that His deeds were accomplished through the power of God. From this standpoint, the mighty deeds of Jesus were the product of God's power that flowed through Him. His powers were charismatic, the result of His having become a channel of the power of God's Spirit.

As people who seek to follow Jesus' example, we, too, are to be channels of God's power. The power of the Spirit is available to us. Within the context of a seriously ill individual, this power means a willingness to provide support to the person, the family, and the health care professionals involved in caring for the person. We will also need the Spirit's strength when we become the patient. An ethic of compassion recognizes that there is a limit to our ability to cure, but that there is no limit to our caring. An ethic of compassion seeks to be with a person through every aspect of suffering, dying, and the accompanying grief that his or her loved ones experience. This is the heart of Christian compassion: not to always provide an answer but to be a presence in the same way in which Jesus was a presence of God's love.

Consider, for example, the story of Job, which we find in the Old Testament. Job was hit with double trouble—personal affliction caused by serious illness, combined with the loss of his many possessions and his family. In the midst of this great suffering, Job's friends came. "They sat with him on the ground seven days and seven nights, and no one spoke a word to him, for they saw that his suffering was very great" (Job 2:13). Imagine the comfort this brought to Job, to have friends who cared so much that they were willing to simply be a silent presence of support even though there was nothing they could "do" to alleviate his serious illness or sense of personal loss. His friends were willing to do something very important—to be fully present with their friend in the face of great suffering.

The willingness to sit with someone and not be able to do anything else, especially to sit with one who is unable to communicate, is the challenge of being a compassionate Christian person. It is truly expressing the love of God through the ministry of presence. It reflects the essence of the incarnation of Jesus Christ. Through the incarnation, God became fully present with us, to show us God's intention for all of humankind.

Concept of Common Sense

There are certain shared experiences that most people understand. All people, for instance, know that life is finite, that love is good and brings happiness, and that hate is evil and brings destruction. This shared background of experience influences the way in which we interact with others on every level of human experience. These shared experiences are the common sense view of the world. The concept of common sense is important in evaluating decisions to limit life-sustaining treatment.

Common sense informs us that if a person is in extreme pain from terminal cancer, he or she should receive whatever pain medication is necessary to relieve the pain. Common sense indicates that futile medical treatments that provide no benefit to the patient are not required and are not ethically justifiable. To continue to keep a brain-dead patient on a ventilator because a family member cannot accept the death of a loved one, for example, serves no useful purpose. If treatment provides no gain, then common sense would call on us to let the patient die in a dignified way.

Common sense also tells us that death is a natural part of the human condition. Death is part of life and should not be viewed as the enemy or an evil to overcome. We must work to regain an understanding of death that respects this aspect of existence with the same awe and reverence with which we respect birth. Just as we hold to the sanctity of life, Christian people should affirm the sanctity of death.

The Roman Catholics have a simple prayer for the sick. They ask God "for a speedy recovery or a happy death." This clearly places the emphasis in the proper place—to cure whenever possible and, when that is no longer possible, to provide comfort and the presence of Jesus Christ until the end. The Presbyterian Church has spoken of this common sense approach to sickness and death in this way:

> The biomedical implications of the theology of death and eternal life reflected in contemporary theologians are several. (1) We fight with God against the power of death;

(2) we hope for a time in history when disease and untimely death will be overcome; (3) we accept death as a part of life experience; (4) we do not live under the dominion of death but live toward the promise of life; (5) we trust the details to God; and (6) in life and death we are with God. . . . There is the danger and temptation to idolize bodily life by making retention of physical life the only good and primary goal. . . . It is indeed idolatrous to try and keep a person's body alive no matter how empty that life may be. Human beings are transcendent creatures. Real life comes from beyond bodily function.[5]

We also find this approach to the sanctity of life and death in Paul's letter to the church in Rome.

We do not live to ourselves, and we do not die to ourselves. If we live, we live to the Lord, and if we die, we die to the Lord; so then, whether we live or whether we die, we are the Lord's. For to this end Christ died and lived again, so that he might be Lord of both the dead and the living. . . . For I am convinced that neither death, nor life, nor angels, nor rulers, nor things present, nor things to come, nor powers, nor height, nor depth, nor anything else in all creation, will be able to separate us from the love of God in Christ Jesus our Lord. (Rom. 14:7–9; 8:38–39)

These passages make it clear that, for the Christian, death is a passage into the eternal presence of God's love. Death is not to be feared but to be faced with a calm confidence and a trust in the sure and certain hope of the resurrection of Jesus Christ.

It would be useful to incorporate the concepts of compassion and common sense, which are derived from Christian theology, into the way we approach treatment decisions. Compassion would cause us to care in ways we have not thought possible before. Common sense would allow us to move in the direction of not providing futile treatments that provide no gain for the patient.

For Christian people, compassion and common sense take place within the context of Jesus' ministry—the One who was the unique, definitive channel of God's love and is our model for all we do. The compassion and common sense of Jesus' ministry can influence positively the current medical model widely in use, which views illness solely in terms of this disease or that syndrome. Jesus' approach was to consider the well-being of the *whole* person, not just the person's illness. If we take this approach seriously, we will be concerned about the quality of both the life and the death of each person.

We need to recapture the importance of theology in discussions and practice concerning life-sustaining treatment. Theology provides a context for our lives and gives our lives ultimate meaning in relationship with God. Theology can provide a level of caring compassion and concern that cannot be found in purely secular approaches to bioethics.

CHAPTER 10

Some Thoughts for Patients and Care Givers

We seldom realize the profound truth of the statement, "When you have your health, you have everything," until we or someone we care about becomes ill. "Good health" is a by-product of a lifestyle that balances the physical, spiritual, and emotional aspects of who we are as human beings. If any aspect of who we are is out of sync, it will eventually affect other parts of our lives. Illness, especially serious illness, can be physically debilitating as well as emotionally and spiritually draining. When we are physically ill or care for someone who is, our lives are out of balance and the resulting stress can be difficult to deal with. So when physical illness strikes, it becomes even more important for us to take care of our spiritual and emotional well-being.

Part of caring for our spiritual and emotional well-being is facing death honestly in an atmosphere of community. Facing death, that of a loved one or our own, is much more of a challenge in our age of modern technology than it was at the beginning of this century. At the beginning of the century, death usually occurred in the home, with friends and family nearby to provide support. The entire family, from grandmother to the smallest child, viewed death as the natural end of life.

Today, the situation has changed. One of the most troublesome aspects of dying at this time is that dying all too often occurs out of context, out of community. Many people die in the isolation of hospital rooms, surrounded by technology that provides medical care but not the caring support of human touch.

Facing Death in an Honest, Healthy Way

We need to regain a sense of the place of death within our lives. We have to consider the limits of medical care and to accept that someday we will die. We need to recapture the attitude that shows all members of the family that death is the natural end of life. Illness and death should take place within the same context as the rest of our lives—among family and friends, in the midst of meaningful activities, in the midst of the most important power in life—love. Patients and family members alike need physical, spiritual, and emotional support when facing illness and death.

Throughout Scripture, we see the attitude that death is simply part of life. We read in Psalm 90:10 that:

The days of our life are seventy years,
or perhaps eighty, if we are strong;
even then their span is only toil and trouble;
they are soon gone, and we fly away.

This knowledge should not cause distress. Rather, it should provide great comfort. In Psalm 89:48, we read, "Who can live and never see death?" In Genesis 25:8, we find a beautiful description of Abraham's death: "Abraham breathed his last and died in a good old age, an old man and full of years, and was gathered to his people."

Jesus' death and resurrection as told in Scripture provide hope for us. God's act of raising Jesus from the dead is a promise to all humankind that when we die we can continue to have an ongoing relationship of love with God and with our loved ones. Scripture assures us that we will never be separated from love—from the love of God or from the love of family and friends.

No matter which illnesses or life-threatening circumstances may beset us, we each have a universal need during times of illness for human interaction, touch, and love. So when we become ill, it is important that we reach out for help. We need to remember the strength we can receive from our faith, family, and friends. When the physical aspect of who we are is weakened, we need to bolster the spiritual and emotional parts of our lives in order to receive the healing that comes from a balanced life.

Making the Most of the Life We Have

Woody Allen once remarked, "I do not want to achieve immortality through my work, I want to achieve immortality by not dying." I am certain that most of us would concur with Woody's reasoning, but we are well aware that this is not possible. We have been created in God's image with almost limitless possibilities to create within the framework of our finite humanity, which will one day come to an end through death. We gain meaning in our existence by doing as much as we can with what God has given us, by living each day to the fullest. In the words of the creed, we are to "glorify God and enjoy God forever." At times, sickness, suffering, and the process of dying make the process of actually living life fully a challenge. Thus we need to consider ways of dealing with illness that encourage healing and wholeness.

When we face illness, we should remember that each of us is like the hub of a spoked wheel. We are at its center; the spokes that go out may be compared to the people and things that are part of our lives—our physician, family members, friends, our spiritual faith, our fears, our hopes, our dreams. If the spokes are damaged or broken, the wheel will not be in balance and won't move smoothly. When the spokes are connected properly and are tight, the wheel will move freely and in balance. This type of harmony—the balance of the spokes and hub—is what health is all about. Let's consider how body, mind, and spirit can work together in interdependence to promote harmony and healing.

Body

During the last fifty years, physicians have become technicians of our bodies. They know body systems backward and forward and can measure virtually every function with exacting precision. We usually go to the doctor when we have a problem with our bodies. Until recently, most of us believed that the physician always knew best. Now we are realizing that medicine is more effective in promoting healing when the physician/patient relationship is viewed as a partnership rather than a paternalistic relationship.

No one, for example, knows your body better than you do. You know what you feel and when you feel it. So "listening" to our bodies when we are sick is an essential element of maintaining our health. Communicating exactly what we feel is wrong with us is essential to an effective doctor/patient relationship. When we listen to our bodies, we are better able to communicate correct information to a physician who can help us become healthy again. In some cases, this will take time to fully explain, so physicians as well as patients must take the time to communicate effectively to ensure that both the physician and the patient understand the complaint and recommended treatment.

Mind

Recently there has been a renewed interest in the relationship between healing and the mind. Bill Moyers completed an excellent public television study on this topic in early 1993. Although the mind can help restore wholeness to the entire person, we cannot simply "think" ourselves well. Conversely, we are not responsible for our own illness because of how we use our minds. However, our minds are powerful tools that can assist our bodies in healing. Consider these examples of using our minds to promote our good health.

Humor. In Proverbs 17:22, we read that laughter is good medicine: "A cheerful heart is a good medicine, but a downcast spirit dries up the bones." Norman Cousins has written about the power of humor in healing, in his book *Anatomy of an Illness*. When we laugh, good things happen in our bodies; when we are mad or angry, bad things happen.

For example, after President Reagan was shot and was being wheeled into surgery, he supposedly said something like, "I hope none of the doctors is a Democrat." One surgeon is said to have replied, "Today we are all Republicans, Mr. President."

Reagan knew that if he lightened up the mood, it would help put people at ease. Laughter helps the body enhance healing.

Love. Karl Menninger said, "Love cures people, both the ones who give it and the ones who receive it." Sometimes we carry unfinished business in our lives—an old grudge or old wound from the past. If we seek to practice the discipline of love, we can begin to bring healing to old wounds and to learn how our past hurts can make us stronger. Especially when we are ill, we need the love and support of special people in our lives.

Imagination. We are all well aware that our creativity resides in our imaginations. We conceive of something "in our mind's eye," for example, before we put brush to canvas or pen to paper. This creative center of our minds can also help us to see our illness differently.

In his book *Love, Miracles, and Medicine*, Dr. Bernie Siegel talks about using the creative aspect of our minds in guided imagery to promote healing for cancer patients. Children he has worked with sometimes even draw pictures of "good cells" eating or destroying the "bad" cancer cells. By explaining in detail what will happen during a surgical procedure, Dr. Siegel has helped patients use their imagination to control bleeding and speed recovery time. Likewise, if we know what to expect and can prepare for a medical procedure, it will be easier for our bodies to respond in ways that promote healing. We can seek to focus on the possibilities and not the limitations of illness, and, in doing so, assist our bodies to make the best of less-than-perfect situations.

Spirit

We can no longer ignore the spiritual dimensions related to illness, death, and dying. This was proven recently by Dr. Melvin Morse, a pediatrician and author of the book *Closer to the Light, Learning from the Near-Death Experiences of Children.* Dr. Morse has conducted scientific studies that confirm that near-death experiences are real occurrences, not hallucinations. Although people from all walks of life have had these experiences, important similarities commonly surface: a being of light; people of light; and a life review. The consistent element running through these experiences is the feeling of a caring and all-loving presence. Dr. Morse concludes that we need to pay close attention to the spiritual dimensions of who we are. He advises us to pay close attention to the pre-death visions of terminally ill patients and not to dismiss them as being unreal. We need to listen carefully to patients and to our own hearts when we experience such happenings.

Dreams. Dreams are real and are an important part of the spiritual aspect of who we are as human beings created in the image of God. People have told me about having dreams of a relative who recently passed away that were as real as anything a person could experience while being "awake." We need to pay attention to our dreams and discern what meaning they may have as we seek healing and wholeness in our lives. The Bible relates a number of examples of people who experienced the presence of God in the context of dream experiences.

Depending on Scripture and Prayer

Illness and death remind us of our complete dependence on God. In these situations, we can discover the power and comfort present in reading Scripture and praying together. Scripture reminds us, for example, that even Paul had an ongoing infirmity. He prayed and prayed that God would provide healing for him. God, in turn, told him, 'My grace is sufficient for you, for power is made perfect in weakness' (2 Cor. 12:9). Sometimes when we feel God's absence in the midst of illness, we need to meditate on the Lord's answer to Paul, to prayerfully consider how God might use our weakness to fulfill God's will.

The psalms are also a great source of strength for people in the midst of adversity. We can clearly see God's healing power in the psalms. In the psalms, people wrestled with God. Consider Psalm 73, where the writer questions why the wicked prosper while good people suffer:

> For I was envious of the arrogant;
>   I saw the prosperity of the wicked.
> For they have no pain;
>   their bodies are sound and sleek.
>
> They set their mouths against heaven,
>   and their tongues range over the earth.
> Therefore the people turn and praise them,
>   and find no fault in them.
> And they say, "How can God know?
>   Is there knowledge in the Most High?"
> Such are the wicked;
>   always at ease, they increase in riches.
> All in vain I have kept my heart clean
>   and washed my hands in innocence. (vv. 3–4, 9–13)

Such questions raised in the psalms capture the universal questions of the human condition. The psalms remind us that we are part of the human family and that all of us, at one time or another, experience hardship, suffering, and illness.

Prayer is important during times of illness. Even when we may not know exactly how to speak to God, it is important for us to share our deepest feelings. God desires this honest sharing, and sharing the secret longings of our hearts will bring us closer to God. Staying in touch with God is very important because without the spiritual dimension of life, life is not complete. We need to work to put the spiritual dimension of healing back into our methods of dealing with illness, dying, and death. We need to remember that Scripture promises that even though our bodies will eventually die, the love we share with each other will live on.

Providing Support for Care Givers

Few things are more difficult than watching a loved one who is stricken with a serious illness or life-threatening situation. Supporting a loved one under these circumstances can be a gut-wrenching experience and an emotional roller coaster. Our tendency is to pull back, to distance ourselves from the person because we feel helpless in the face of illness. We want to avoid situations that make us acknowledge our own mortality.

Yet it's extremely important to stay in touch with the seriously ill person. The involvement of family and friends can be a tremendous support.

During illness, family members may be able to play a vital role. All of us feel most comfortable in our own homes rather than in hospital rooms. Family members often can be instrumental in seeking ways for patients to receive ongoing home health care for chronic illness.

Although home health care can be difficult for a family to provide, there are more and more home health care agencies available to support families in this effort. Many communities have Visiting Nursing Associations that provide licensed health care workers who visit and monitor a patient's progress. With proper help, the family can provide tremendous support for a chronically ill patient by enabling him or her to stay at home in familiar surroundings.

Friends of the patient and family can be a great emotional boost in the midst of illness. Often the isolation that accompanies illness can bring feelings of depression or dread. Some studies have shown that when a patient is very sick even the number of his or her physician's visits drops dramatically.

A friend of mine who was eighty-six years old and recently died of liver cancer was one of the fortunate few who had a different experience. During the last three months of his life, he received care at home with the help of a home health care agency. Right up until the end, his many friends stopped in for short visits to let him know they cared. In this type of situation, the family and patient need to draw on support from health care professionals as well as friends so that they may face death in ways that can bring peace to all concerned.

Resources for Family Care Givers

We all need the support of others when we are dealing with difficult aspects of life. This is especially true when we are providing care for a loved one who is ill. Family members should seek support often in order to find the strength to carry on. Although authors have written entire books on support for family care givers, let's look at two ways in which families of chronically ill patients can find the support they need.

Family members should seek out professional resources in their community. If a family is going to attempt to provide care for a chronically ill family member at home, support for physical care will be needed. Arrangements can be made for almost every aspect of medical care. Often the best place to begin is with a home health care agency that can provide necessary medical care. The discharge planner at an acute care hospital can provide information on a suitable home health care agency.

Usually the home health care agency will send out a social worker to do an "intake assessment," which means discovering the patient's medical needs and what type of assistance the family needs in order to provide appropriate care for the patient. This assessment gives family members a prime opportunity to discuss concerns about the patient's actual health care. The agency can coordinate needed health care, which in most cases can be provided entirely in the patient's home.

In addition to physical support, family members need to find their own emotional support system. Some family members may wish to seek the support of a religious professional; others may feel comfortable talking in a group setting. Many hospitals provide support group meetings for families. These meetings, organized through the hospitals' pastoral care departments, often have no set agenda. People simply share their feelings, fears, frustrations, and all the additional emotional baggage that goes along with taking care of a chronically ill loved one. This act of catharsis—sharing deeply held feelings—can be a healing experience for family members as they seek to support and care for their loved ones.

CHAPTER 11

Some Thoughts for Pastoral Care Givers and Religious Professionals

The role of the religious care giver is essential when patients and their families face a serious illness or imminent death. One of the greatest challenges for any person, including religious professionals, is to provide true understanding and support for a dying patient. In order to give the support needed, the pastoral care giver needs to cultivate that "special sense" which enables him or her to minister effectively to everyone involved. Patients and families also need support from physicians at this time. But when medical technology has exhausted its abilities on behalf of the patient, the pastoral care giver can offer solace and access to the spiritual realm of human existence. And when medical technology runs out, those are the only answers.

Consider how one sensitive person views the doctor-patient relationship as the time of death approaches:

I understand now that the process of death can release overwhelming emotions not only in patients but also in physicians. Physicians may not be prepared to handle the situation either as physicians or as bystanders. Perhaps, as a result of their education and conditioning, physicians are afraid to feel helpless and to project hopelessness to their patients.

Although physicians know that knowledge and technology do not always control human diseases, most feel that it is their responsibility to keep patients alive, almost unconditionally. . . . So they [physicians] must begin to see how important it is for them to participate with the terminally ill patient in the process of death. The dying person needs to feel that he or she has not lost meaning for those who are close, one of whom is inevitably the doctor who has tried so hard to cure the patient. With death close, dying patients may still want to express what they experience and to convey their fantasies about death. The presence of the doctor in this last phase of life may be crucial for a peaceful death. It can allow the patient not only to die with self-respect but also to feel less lonely.[1]

Pastoral care givers and religious professionals can and should provide similar support to dying patients and others who are involved in the bedside vigil.

For instance, one important role the pastoral care giver can fulfill is to be a bridge between health care professionals, the patient, and the realm of the perceived unknown. When death is near, the pastoral care giver serves as a link to the place of the presence of our loving God, who ultimately controls life and death. Often when medical interventions have ceased to be useful to the patient and all that is left to do is wait until death comes, the clergy care giver can coordinate a vigil to bring strength and comfort to dying people and their families.

Before becoming deeply involved in the lives of patients and their families, however, religious professionals should be sure such a ministry will not unduly or negatively affect their well-being. Being a supportive care giver to people involved in the intense emotional experiences of facing death takes a heavy toll. Care givers are human, too, having all the same feelings, doubts, and questions as any other person involved in the care of the dying. So it is important that each care giver have a support network where he or she can be nurtured as well. With that point in mind, let's look at three objectives that religious care givers have when a patient is dying.

1. *Maintain physical contact with the patient.* The primary responsibility in providing care to the dying patient is to respond to his or her needs for caring companionship. Since a dying patient is often unable to communicate, it is important to be present in such a way that the patient knows he or she is not alone. This can be accomplished by occasionally holding the patient's hand and by speaking so the patient knows someone who cares is near.

2. *Meet the needs of close family members.* Equally important to maintaining contact with the patient is the responsibility to respond to the needs of family members. Here the religious care giver must use what I call the "special sense." This special sense is honed by experience but must be accompanied by knowledge as well. The special sense is a gift that brings insight into how to minister effectively to loved ones who gather at the patient's bedside. This insight may signal that the moment is ripe for prayer, a word of comfort from the Scriptures, or simply a time for silence.

3. *Support health care professionals.* In addition to comforting terminally ill or life-sustained patients

and their families, the religious care giver can use
the "special sense" to bring comfort to the health
care professionals involved. Nursing and level-of-
care staff often have the closest relationship to the
patient. During the hours immediately preceding
death, they are often burdened with the chores of
charting, administering medication, and taking
care of official business.

When the patient dies, health care professionals can be
exhausted and emotionally spent. The sensitive pastoral care
giver will therefore seek to be a sounding board for health
care professionals, a person with whom they can talk, weep,
and share the experience of death.

Being with people when they die is a life-changing
experience because every life is a precious gift from God, and
the experience inevitably confronts all present with their
own mortality. The actual moment of death is a mystery as
profound and powerful as the moment of birth.

Practical Ways to Help Dying Patients and Their Families

Dr. Sharon Mass has written a useful piece on caring for
the dying from a social service perspective. Entitled "A Crisis
Intervention Model for Dying Patients and Their Families,"[2]
it provides care givers with five important and practical ways
to help dying patients and their families:

1. *Communicate effectively.* If the patient is able,
    communication is a paramount need for both the
    patient and the family. Although listening offers
    direct comfort and support, the intensity of feel-

ings evoked by dying and death engender nonverbal communication, too. Intense emotional communication, in turn, facilitates emotional healing for terminal patients. With appropriate emotional support, patients and their families can focus on pressing issues as well as plan for the future.

2. *Be a knowledgeable clinician.* The pastoral care giver must be knowledgeable about the process of dying, defense and coping mechanisms, and various medical treatments. By educating patients and their families about what they might experience emotionally and by translating medical terminology into lay terms, the care giver acts as an advocate for patients and helps them sort out the real from the unreal.

3. *Empower the patient.* It is important to encourage dying patients to retain authority and control over daily tasks and decision making to the longest extent possible. For as long as possible, patients should be allowed to retain autonomy, a sense of identity, and self-esteem. Sometimes the silent presence of a care giver offers more support for patients and their families than does "helping" activity. When no more can be done or said, simply holding the patient's hands or shedding tears will help the patient let go of life.

4. *Prepare the family.* Often the pastoral care giver must act as an interpreter and mediator, clarifying what family members know, sensing why they may be angry or withdrawn, and finding out how they perceive their own situations and the actions of others. The task of the care giver is to assist the families in anticipating and preparing for separation from their loved ones.

5. *Facilitate grieving.* Physicians through the ages have suspected that grief is a significant cause of sickness and death. Family members who assist their dying relatives must be considered to be victims and eventually patients who need as much caring support as the dying person. A severe loss makes life seem empty. A grieving person's ability to overcome grief depends on the support available as well as the development of a renewed self-esteem and sense of meaning. Loss, if mourned successfully, strengthens and enhances the ego, thus serving as an important aspect of development. The goal of grief work is to help people release their emotions so that they can relinquish ties to their loved ones.

Barbara Hills LesStrang, in her book *Afterloss: A Recovery Companion for Those Who Are Grieving* describes the pain of loss with vivid accuracy:

And as we pace from room to room, our wounds still raw, our chests heavy with aching hearts, that empty chair, that symbol of bereavement, sits there, mockingly, a daily reminder affirming our loss and our anguish. The empty chair is a silent symbol that our lives will never, ever be the same again.[3]

LesStrang makes it clear that the only way for healing to begin after a loss is to place yourself in the empty chair and begin, in your own way, to confront the threatening dangers and explore long-held fears and feelings of abandonment. When these powerful feelings of loss are confronted head-on with the help of prayer and Scripture, healing will begin in God's way at God's time. Let's look at how religious care givers can provide spiritual support to patients and their families as death approaches.

Spiritual Support for Patients and Their Families

The religious care giver who serves on the health care team can also provide important spiritual support at the difficult moment of death.

Prayers

A number of prayers have been written that may be used with families when a life-support system is turned off. These prayers can easily be adapted for personal or family use. The following sample prayer that I wrote could be used when life-sustaining medical treatment will be withdrawn.

> *Minister: Let us unite our hearts together in prayer. Loving God, we are mindful that You are the Creator of all life.*
>
> **Family:** *Gracious Lord, help us to put our trust in Your promise of eternal life.*
>
> *Minister: Merciful God, You promise us in Your Word that nothing will separate us from Your love we know in Jesus Christ.*
>
> **Family:** *Precious Lord, death is difficult to understand, but help us to see that You are always with us.*
>
> *Minister: Giver of all good things, we give You our heartfelt thanks for the gift of _____ (name) _____.*
>
> **Family:** *Loving Spirit, help us to remember all the love we received from _____, the good times and the lessons learned, as we remove this treatment and allow him/her to return to Your presence.*
>
> *Minister: Merciful God, we now humbly pray that You allow Your servant to depart in peace. Let us now do what needs to be done to release _____ (name) into the hope we have through Jesus' resurrection.*
>
> **Family:** *Amen. Lord God, we trust in Your promises, and we pray for the comfort of the Holy Spirit as we face the pain of our loss. Thank You for Your love and grace and goodness toward us.*

Although this is an excellent example of a prayer that might be appropriate when a patient is dying, it is also important that the pastoral care giver in any situation be sensitive to the needs of the family members. Rather than using a prepared prayer, it may be more appropriate for the religious care giver to say a prayer that incorporates elements of the above prayer. The prayer should be tailored to the unique situation of that particular family. This will again require use of the care giver's "special sense" in order to speak a word from the Lord that will bring the comfort of God's Holy Spirit.

The Psalms

In the same way that prayer can bring comfort to the family and friends, Scripture can also bring comfort. The psalms are especially helpful in this regard. Many of them speak of God's steadfast love in the midst of life's hardships. The Psalter is filled with deep emotions—emotions that are similar to those the family of a dying patient experiences. The soul-searching so clearly stated in the psalms provides a rich source of material on which religious care givers can draw when seeking to comfort people who are confronting death. (The psalms can also be used as a place where religious care givers can begin their own personal spiritual journey.)

As a deer longs for flowing streams,
   so my soul longs for you, O God.
My soul thirsts for God,
   for the living God.
When shall I come and behold
   the face of God?
My tears have been my food
   day and night,
while people say to me continually,
   "Where is your God?"
These things I remember,
   as I pour out my soul:

how I went with the throng,
   and led them in procession to the house of God,

with glad shouts and songs of thanksgiving,
    a multitude keeping festival.
Why are you cast down, O my soul,
    and why are you disquieted within me?
Hope in God; for I shall again praise him,
    my help and my God. (Ps. 42:1–5a)

In this psalm, the psalmist reveals his deep longing for God. At the beginning of the prayer, he pleads for God's presence in the midst of some trouble, possibly physical illness. Even in the midst of such distress, he remembers God's goodness, and how He led the people in a procession of shouts of joy and thanksgiving. The remembrance of God's steadfast love and abundant joy enables the psalmist to hope even in the midst of adversity. This psalm powerfully demonstrates that God is with us through every aspect of life, including serious illness and the dying process. A prayer such as the following one I have written could be based on this psalm:

> Gracious Lord of all our comings and goings, we turn our hearts' full attention to You at this difficult time. We pray for Your loving presence, the joy and courage that sustain us. Please grant _____ Your peace. Help us to remember Your blessings. Empower us with Your hope. We thank You for Your love, which never leaves us alone. Strengthen us, Lord, we humbly pray. Amen.

Psalm 46 is a prayer that declares God's presence with us during all the circumstances we encounter in life. Here the psalmist clearly communicates that God provides both solace and courage to face life's adversities. Let's look at verses 1–3 and 11:

God is our refuge and strength,
  a very present help in trouble.
Therefore we will not fear, though the earth should change,
  though the mountains shake in the heart of the sea;
though its waters roar and foam,
  though the mountains tremble with its tumult.

The LORD of hosts is with us;
  the God of Jacob is our refuge.

In the midst of the changes we all experience in life, there is one constant: the steadfast love of God. God will give us strength and comfort as we face illness or death. God is always with us to help us. If we call on Him, God will never leave us alone. I've written the following prayer based on Psalm 46:

Merciful God, we give You thanks that Your love for us is an everlasting love, a love that never lets us go. In the midst of our trouble here, Lord, we ask for Your courage and Your peace. Empower us by Your Holy Spirit to be faithful to You.

Quiet our hearts so we may hear Your voice of forgiveness, love, and peace. We are thankful that You are always with us. Be with us now, we humbly pray. Amen.

The protection of the Lord is greater than any threat we may encounter. "And remember," Jesus says in Matthew 28:20, "I am with you always, to the end of the age." And in John 14, Jesus tells His disciples that He will prepare a place for them in heaven. God's presence is continual. When there is a threat from evil or temptation, God is nearby when we call out. Psalm 121 also speaks in a powerful way that God is our help and protection:

I lift up my eyes to the hills—
   from where will my help come?
My help comes from the LORD,
   who made heaven and earth.
He will not let your foot be moved;
   he who keeps you will not slumber.
He who keeps Israel
   will neither slumber nor sleep.
The LORD is your keeper;
   the LORD is your shade at your right hand.
The sun shall not strike you by day,
   nor the moon by night.
The LORD will keep you from all evil;
   he will keep your life.
The LORD will keep
   your going out and your coming in
from this time on and forevermore.

Again, the religious care giver can write a prayer, such as the following, based on Psalm 121:

Loving God, we pray for our friend, _____. You, Lord, are aware of _____'s illness. You know how much pain the family feels. Surround this family with Your loving presence. Grant them the help and courage they need at this difficult time. Sustain them now by Your Holy Spirit. We thank You for watching over us all the days of our lives. Bless us now, we humbly pray. Amen.

These are just a few examples of how the psalms can provide a great source of strength and comfort to individuals and families facing serious illness and death. Pastoral care givers should encourage terminally ill people and their family members to write their own psalms, to express deep emotions through this process. Patients, family members, and friends should also be encouraged to explore their feelings through prayer, just as the psalmist did. This process can help to keep communication with God open during a time when some people only want to curse God.

The Value of Hospice Care

Hospice care is another resource from which religious care givers can gain insight into effective ministry to dying patients and their families. The hospice philosophy is important. This unique part of the health care system exists not to postpone death but, through special skills and therapies, to help the patient and the patient's family live as fully as possible until death occurs. The intention of hospice is to affirm life through supportive care.

The goals of hospice care are receiving increased recognition. These goals include the provision of a dignified, comfortable death for terminally ill patients and the care of patients and their families as a unit. Another goal of hospice care is to control terminally ill patients' pain and other symptoms and to help patients and family members deal with the psychological issues and family concerns they face. Hospice emphasizes care which will enhance patients' quality of life rather than seeking to cure disease or extend life. Pain control, not only physical pain but "total pain"—mental, physical, social, and spiritual—is also addressed.

I believe we can learn much from the hospice model. This model of mutual sharing, caring, celebrating, and rejoicing at the end of life can teach us important lessons on how we should live our lives. The value of hospice can be seen in its holistic approach. Patients are not viewed as isolated persons who have diseases. Rather, patients are viewed within the context of the human relationships that give meaning to life. An interdisciplinary team provides care to patients and their families.

Hospice also encourages patients who are able to stay at home during the dying process to do so. In these cases, the family becomes the primary care giver, and professionals visit to maintain pain control. Motivated by compassion and common sense, the hospice approach clearly focuses on the overall needs of dying patients and their families.

Health care professionals such as physicians, nurses, social workers, and chaplains should receive formal training in the hospice philosophy and additional training in caring for the terminally ill and their families. This would lead to more humane care for dying people throughout the health care system, and would increase the role of hospice care in helping patients and their families.

Death is part of life, part of God's plan. With God's help, we can face this final stage of growth with calm confidence. Bioethical dilemmas can be resolved through a consistent and systematic application of ethical and theological principles. The resolution of these dilemmas must include compassion and common sense. By documenting our personal values, we will spare our loved ones and health care professionals from having to second-guess the treatment we would want if we were unable to decide for ourselves.

Appendix A

DURABLE POWER OF ATTORNEY FOR HEALTH CARE/PROXY DIRECTIVE

I, [Full Name]_____, residing at Address _____
City _____ State _____ Zip _____, appoint as my Agent (attorney-in-fact): [Agent's Full Name] _____, of [His/Her Address] _____.

City _____ State _____ Zip _____
Telephone Number _____

If my Agent is unwilling or unable to serve, then I appoint as my alternate Agent (attorney-in-fact): [Alternate Agent's Full Name] _____,of [Address] _____.

City _____ State _____ Zip _____.
Telephone Number _____

My Agent shall have the authority to make health care decisions for me, subject to any limitations I state below, if I am unable to make decisions for myself. My Agent's authority becomes effective if it is confirmed in writing, by two physicians, that I lack the capacity to make or to communicate informed health care decisions. My Agent is then to have the same authority to make health care decisions as I would if I had the capacity to make them, except: [here list the limitations, if any, you wish to place on your Agent's authority]: _____

_____.

I direct my Agent to make decisions based upon my Agent's understanding of my personal values. If my personal values are unknown, my Agent is to make decisions on the basis of his/her assessment of my best interests. Photocopies of this Durable Power of Attorney for Health Care/Proxy Instructive shall have the same force and effect as the original.

Signed [Your Name]_____

Date   _____

WITNESS STATEMENT

We, the undersigned, declare under the penalty of perjury that the Declarant who signed this advance directive did so in our presence, and that the Declarant appears to be of sound mind and under no constraints or undue influence. We did not sign the Declarant's signature for or at the direction of the Declarant. We are at least eighteen (18) years of age and are not related to the Declarant by blood or marriage, entitled to any portion of the estate of the Declarant under any will of the Declarant or codicil thereto now existing or by operation of law, or directly financially responsible for the Declarant's medical care. We are not the Declarant's attending physician, an employee of the attending physician, or an employee of the health facility in which the Declarant is a patient. Neither of us is named as the Agent or Alternate Agent in this document.

In our presence this _____ day of _____, 19___.

I sign my name to this advance directive for health care on this _____ day of _____ , 19___.

WITNESS 1

Name [Print] _____

Signature _____

Address _____

City _____ State _____ Zip _____

Telephone Number _____

WITNESS 2

Name [Print] _____

Signature _____

Address _____

City _____ State _____ Zip _____

Telephone Number _____

Use the following if your state requires that this document be acknowledged before a Notary Public:

Before me, _____, on this
[insert name of Notary Public]

_____ day of _____ 19___, personally appeared

_____,[name of Declarant completing this form] known to me to be the

Declarant whose name is signed to the foregoing instrument, and who, in my presence, did subscribe his/her name to the attached Durable Power of Attorney for Health Care/Proxy Directive on this date, and that said Declarant at the time of execution of said Declaration was over the age of eighteen (18) years and of sound mind.

Seal   Notary Public

PHYSICIAN STATEMENT

I, the undersigned, am the physician of _____
_____. I have seen this document and discussed it with _____.
If _____ becomes unable to make competent decisions, I understand that it is my duty to be guided by this advance directive.
Signature_____

COMBINATION DURABLE POWER OF ATTORNEY FOR HEALTH CARE/INSTRUCTIVE DIRECTIVE

I, [Your Name] _____, a citizen
of the State of _____, residing at [Address]
_____, City _____
State _____ Zip _____, Telephone Number
_____ do hereby designate and appoint as my Agent:

Name _____

Address_____

City _____ State _____Zip _____

Telephone Number_____

This person is empowered to make health care decisions for me as authorized in this document. If my Agent is unwilling or unable to serve, then I appoint:

Name_____

Address_____

City _____ State _____Zip _____

Telephone Number _____

as my Alternate Agent, empowered to make health care decisions for me as authorized in this document.

If I become unable to make informed choices concerning my health care, I hereby grant my Agent full power and authority to make health care decisions for me, subject to my preferences and values stated below.

My Agent's authority becomes effective if it is confirmed in writing, by two physicians, that I am unable to make informed choices regarding my health care.

I hereby direct my Agent to make decisions on the basis of his/her understanding of my preferences and values. My Agent should seek to weigh the burdens and benefits of any form of medical treatment and authorize those treatments that provide an overall net gain (where benefits are greater than burdens), and are in my overall best interest. Photocopies of this advance directive shall have the same force and effect as the original.

Statement of Treatment Preferences, Values, and Limitations:

(If you wish, simply attach your completed Values History/Medical Directive.) _____

_____

_____

(Attach additional pages if more space is needed.)

I sign my name to this advance directive for health care on this _____ day of _____, 19___.

Signature of principal:_____

This directive will not be valid unless it is signed by two qualified adult witnesses or acknowledged by a Notary Public.

WITNESS STATEMENT

We, the undersigned, declare under the penalty of perjury that the Declarant who signed this advance directive did so in our presence, and that the Declarant appears to be of sound mind and under no constraints or undue influence. We did not sign the Declarant's signature for or at the direction of the Declarant. We are at least eighteen (18) years of age and are not related to the Declarant by blood or marriage, entitled to any portion of the estate of the Declarant under any will of the Declarant or codicil thereto now existing or by operation of law, or directly financially responsible for the Declarant's medical care. We are not the Declarant's attending physician, an employee of the attending physician, or an employee of the health facility in which the Declarant is a patient. Neither of us is named as the Agent or Alternate Agent in this document.

WITNESS 1

Name _____

Address _____

City_____ State _____ Zip _____

Telephone Number _____

Date _____

Signature _____

WITNESS 2

Name _____

Address _____

City _____ State _____ Zip _____

Telephone Number_____

Date _____

Signature _____

Signature of patient advocate or ombudsman (if needed):

_____

Date_____

CERTIFICATION OF ACKNOWLEDGMENT OF NOTARY PUBLIC

Use the following if your state requires that this document be acknowledged before a Notary Public:

Before me, _____, on this
                  [insert name of Notary Public]

_____ day of _____, 19___, personally appeared
_____,[name of Declarant completing this form] known to me to be the Declarant whose name is signed to the foregoing instrument, and who, in my presence, did subscribe his/her name to the attached Combination Durable Power of Attorney for Health

Care/Instructive Directive on this date, and that said Declarant at the time of execution of said Declaration was over the age of eighteen (18) years and of sound mind.

Seal   Notary Public

PHYSICIAN STATEMENT

I, the undersigned, am the physician of _____
_____. I have seen this document and discussed it with _____.
If_____ becomes unable to make competent decisions, I understand that it is my duty to be guided by this advance directive.
Signature _____

THE LIVING WILL/INSTRUCTIVE DIRECTIVE

Declaration made this _____ day of _____ , 19___.

I, _____, being of sound mind, willfully and voluntarily make known my desires that my dying shall not be artificially prolonged under circumstances set forth below, and do declare:

If I should have an incurable and irreversible condition that has been diagnosed by two physicians and that will result in my death within a relatively short time without the administration of life-sustaining treatment or that has produced an irreversible coma or persistent vegetative state, and I am no longer able to make competent decisions regarding my medical treatment, I direct my physician to withhold or withdraw treatment that only prolongs the process of dying or the irreversible coma or persistent vegetative state I am in and that is not necessary for my comfort or to alleviate pain.

If I should have an incurable or irreversible condition or should be in an irreversible coma or persistent vegetative state, I direct my attending physician to withhold or withdraw artificially administered nutrition and hydration that only prolongs the process of dying.

_____ (Sign here to indicate you would not want tube feeding—artificial nutrition and hydration.)

Declarant's statement of values and treatment preferences

List here any of your treatment preferences or values concerning quality of life, or attach your completed Values History and/or Medical Directive.

_____

_____

_____

In the absence of my ability to give directions regarding the use of such life-sustaining procedures, it is my intention that this declaration shall be honored by my family and physicians as the final expression of my legal right to refuse medical treatment and to accept the consequences of such refusal.

I understand the full import of this declaration, and I am emotionally and mentally competent to make this declaration.

Signed _____

Address _____

City _____ State _____ Zip _____

Telephone Number _____

WITNESS STATEMENT

We, the undersigned, declare under the penalty of perjury that the Declarant who signed this advance directive did so in our presence, and that the Declarant appears to be of sound mind and under no constraints or undue influence.

We did not sign the Declarant's signature for or at the direction of the Declarant. We are at least eighteen (18) years of age and are not related to the Declarant by blood or marriage, entitled to any portion of the estate of the Declarant under any will of the Declarant or codicil thereto now existing or by operation of law, or directly financially responsible for the Declarant's medical care. We are not the Declarant's attending physician, an employee of the attending physician, or an employee of the health facility in which the Declarant is a patient. Neither of us is named as the Agent or Alternate Agent in this document.

Witness (please print)_____

Signature_____

Address _____

City _____ State _____ Zip _____

Telephone Number_____

Witness (please print)_____

Signature_____

Address_____

City _____ State _____ Zip _____

Telephone Number_____

Use the following if your state requires that this document be acknowledged before a Notary Public:

Before me, _____, on this

[insert name of Notary Public]

_____ day of _____ , 19___, personally appeared,

_____

[name of Declarant completing this form] known to me to be the Declarant whose name is signed to the foregoing instrument, and who, in my presence, did subscribe his/her name to the attached Living Will on this date, and that said Declarant at the time of execution of said Declaration was over the age of eighteen (18) years and of sound mind.

Seal   Notary Public

PHYSICIAN STATEMENT

I, the undersigned, am the physician of _____
_____. I have seen this document and discussed it with_____.
If _____ becomes unable to make competent decisions, I understand that it is my duty to be guided by this advance directive.
Signature_____

Appendix B

IMPORTANT NOTICE TO MEDICAL PERSONNEL

_____ has executed an advance directive. If I am unable to make my own health decisions, then those providing for my care should be guided by this document. If I have designated a person to make decisions on my behalf, the names of those persons are on this card. My physician has a copy of my directive.

········· [Fold Here] ·········

Agent's name _____

Work phone _____

Home phone _____

Alternate _____

phone _____

Physician _____

phone _____

Selected Bibliography

Abrams, Natalie, and Michael Buckner, eds. *Medical Ethics: A Clinical Textbook and Reference for the Health Care Professions.* Cambridge, Massachusetts: MIT Press, 1983.

Atkins, Gary M. "Theological History of Catholic Teaching on Prolonging Life." In *Moral Responsibility In Prolonging Life Decisions,* eds. Donald G. McCarthy and Albert S. Moraczewski. St. Louis: Pope John XXIII Center, 1981.

Barnum, Barbara. "Can Healers Make Their Peace With Death?" *Healthweek* 4, no. 13 (July 16, 1990): 19.

Barry, Robert. "Feeding the Comatose and the Common Good in the Catholic Tradition." *The Thomist* 53 no. 1: 1-30.

Barth, Karl. "Respect for Life" and "The Protection of Life." In *Church Dogmatics III/4.* Edinburgh: T. and T. Clark, 1961.

Baskett, Peter J. F. "The Ethics of Resuscitation." *British Medical Journal* (July 1986).

Beauchamp, Tom and James Childress. *Principles of Biomedical Ethics.* 2nd ed. New York: Oxford University Press, 1983.

Boly, William. "Choices of the Heart." *Hippocrates* 40 (May/June 1988).

Borg, Marcus J. *Jesus, A New Vision: Spirit, Culture, and the Life of Discipleship.* Harper and Row, 1987.

Engelhardt, H. Tristram. "Bioethics and the Process of Embodiment." *Perspectives in Biology and Medicine* 18 (Summer 1975): 486-500.

Engelhardt, H. Tristram. "Medicine and the Concept of Person." In *Ethical Issues in Death and Dying,* eds. Tom L. Beauchamp and Seymour Perlin. Englewood Cliffs, New Jersey: Prentice-Hall, 1978.

Englehardt, H. Tristram. *The Foundations of Bioethics.* New York: Oxford University Press, 1986.

Fletcher, Joseph. "Ethics and Euthanasia." *American Journal of Nursing* 73 (1973): 671.

Fletcher, Joseph. "The Right to Die: A Theologian's Comment." *Atlantic Monthly* (April 1968): 62-63.

Forguson, Lynd. *Common Sense.* London: Routledge, 1989.

Francoeur, Robert T. *Biomedical Ethics: A Guide to Decision Making.* New York: John Wiley & Sons, 1983.

Frankena, William K. "Deontological Theories." In *Contemporary Issues in Bioethics,* 2nd ed., eds. Tom L. Beauchamp and LeRoy Walters. Belmont, California: Wadsworth Publishing Company, 1982.

Gustafson, James M. *The Contribution of Theology to Medical Ethics.* Milwaukee: Marquette University Press, 1975.

Gustafson, James M. "Ethics From a Theocentric Perspective". *Ethics and Theology, Vol. II.* Chicago: University of Chicago Press, 1984.

Jameton, Andrew. *Nursing Practice: The Ethical Issues.* Englewood Cliffs, New Jersey: Prentice-Hall, 1984.

John Paul II. *Familiaris Consortio.* Washington, D.C.: USCC Publications, 1982.

Kaiser Permanente Hospital. Hospice Program Brochure. 1985.

MacKay, R.D. "Terminating Life, Sustaining Treatment: Recent United States Developments." *Journal of Medical Ethics* 14 (1988): 135-139.

Maguire, Daniel C. "Death and the Moral Domain." *The St. Luke's Journal of Theology* 20 (June 1977): 205-206.

McCarthy, Donald. "Care of Severely Defective Newborn Babies." In *Moral Responsibility in Prolonging Life Decisions*, eds. Donald McCarthy and Albert S. Moraczewski. St. Louis: Pope John XXIII Center, 1981.

McCartney, James J. "Catholic Positions on Withholding Sustenance for the Terminally Ill". The Catholic Health Association of The United States, 1986.

McCormick, Richard. "A Proposal for 'Quality of Life' Criteria for Sustaining Life." *Hospital Progress* 56 (1975): 76.

McCormick, Richard. "Theology and Bioethics." *The Hastings Center Report* (March/April 1989): 5-10.

McCormick, Richard. "Reflections on the Literature." In *Readings in Moral Theology* no. 1: 318-319.

McIntyre, M. "Medicolegal Considerations and Recommendations." *Journal of the American Medical Association* 255, no. 21 (1986): 2979-2984.

O'Rourke, Kevin. "The A.M.A. Statement on Tube Feeding: an Ethical Analysis." *America* (November 22, 1986): 323-327.

Parad, Howard J. and Libbie G. Parad, eds. *Crisis Intervention Book 2: The Practitioner's Sourcebook for Grief Therapy.* Milwaukee: Family Service America, 1990.

Paul VI. "Statement on the International Year of the Child, 1979." *Origins* 8 (July 26, 1978): 120-121.

Pius XII. "Address of the First International Congress of Histopathology of the Nervous System." September 13, 1952.

Pius XII. "The Apostolate of the Sick and Suffering." Address to a group of invalids at the Vatican, 1957. *The Pope Speaks* 4 (1957/58): 399-402.

Pius XII. "The Prolongation of Life." Address to the International Congress of Anesthesiologists, 1957. The Pope Speaks 4 (1957/58): 395-396.

President's Commission for the Study of Ethical Problems in Medicine and Biomedical and Behavioral Research. "Deciding to Forgo Life-Sustaining Treatment: Ethical, Medical, and Legal Issues in Treatment Decisions". Washington, D.C.: U.S. Government Printing Office, 1982.

President's Commission for the Study of Ethical Problems in Medicine and Biomedical and Behavioral Research. "Making Health Care Decisions". Washington, D.C.: U.S. Government Printing Office, 1982.

Ramsey, Paul. *Ethics at the Edge of Life: Medical and Legal Intersections*. New Haven: Yale University Press, 1978.

Ramsey, Paul. "Introduction." In *Infanticide and the Handicapped Newborn*, eds. Dennis J. Horan and Melinda Delahoyde. Provo, Utah: Brigham Young University Press, 1982.

Report of the Joint Committee on Bioethics, San Diego County (May 1989).

Ross, Judith Wilson. *Handbook for Hospital Ethics Committees*. American Hospital Publishing, Inc., 1986.

Seravalli, Egilde P. "The Dying Patient, The Physician, and the Fear of Death." *New England Journal of Medicine* 319 no. 26 (December 29, 1988): 1728-1730.

Shannon, Thomas, and Jo Ann Manfra, eds. *Law and Bioethics: Texts with Commentary on Major U. S. Court Decisions*. New York: Paulist Press, 1982.

Sharp, Earl E., ed. *Theology and Bioethics: Exploring the Foundations and Frontiers*. Dordrecht, Holland: D. Riedel Publishing Company, 1985.

Steinbrook and Lo. "Artificial Feeding: Solid Ground, Not a Slippery Slope." *New England Journal of Medicine* 286 (February 4, 1988): 286-290.

Sundram, Clarence. "Informed Consent for Major Medical Treatment of Mentally Disabled People: A New Approach." *New England Journal of Medicine* 318, no. 21 (May 26, 1988).

Taylor, Humphrey. Correspondence. *New England Journal of Medicine* 322 no. 26 (June 28, 1990): 1891-1892.

The Joint Committee on Bioethics of the Los Angeles County Medical Association and the Los Angeles Bar Association. "Principles and Guidelines Concerning the Foregoing of Life-Sustaining Treatment for Adult Patients". February 1990.

The Hastings Center. "Guidelines on the Termination of Life-Sustaining Treatment and the Care of the Dying". Indiana University Press, 1987.

The Covenant of Life and the Caring Community. Louisville, Kentucky: The Office of the General Assembly, 1983.

The Sacred Congregation for the Doctrine of the Faith, "Euthanasia (Jura et Bona)" in *The Pope Speaks* (May 5, 1980: 289-296).

Notes

Chapter 1: Two Women Who Challenged Our Thinking

1. William Boly, "Choices of the Heart," *Hippocrates* (May/June 1988): 40.
2. Missouri Supreme Court, Ruling in the Case of Cruzan v. Harmon, et al. v. McCanse (November 16, 1988) 760 S. W. 2d 408, 416-17 (Mo. 1988).
3. United States Supreme Court, Ruling in the Case of Cruzan v. Director, Missouri Department of Health, 110 S. Ct. 2841 (1990).

Chapter 2: Making Medical Treatment Decisions

1. J. C. Fletcher and M. L. White, "The Patient Self-Determination Act: On Balance, More Help Than Hindrance," *JAMA* 266, 3 (July 17, 1991): 411. Schloendorff v. Society of New York Hospital, 211 NY, 125, 105 NE 92 (1914).
2. Omnibus Budget Reconciliation Act of 1990. Title IV, Section 4206. *Congressional Record.* October 26, 1990; 136:H12456-H12457.

Chapter 3: Ethical and Theological Foundations

1. Judith Wilson Ross with Sister Corrine Bayley, Vicki Michel, and Deborah Pugh, *Handbook for Hospital Ethics Committees* (Chicago: American Hospital Publishing, Inc., 1986), p. 5.
2. *Guidelines on the Termination of Life-Sustaining Treatment and the Care of the Dying* (Bloomington: Indiana University Press, 1987), p. 2.
   Hereafter referred to as *Guidelines*.
3. Ibid., p. 3.
4. President's Commission for the Study of Ethical Problems in Medicine and Biomedical and Behavioral Research, *Deciding to Forego Life-Sustaining Treatment: Ethical, Medical, and Legal Issues in Treatment Decisions* (New York: Concern for Dying—An Educational Council, 1983), pp. 43-44. Hereafter referred to as President's Commission.

5. "Declaration on Euthanasia." Prepared by the Sacred Congregation for the Doctrine of the Faith (Boston: The Daughters of St. Paul, 1980), pp. 11-12. Hereafter referred to as "Declaration on Euthanasia."

6. President's Commission, p. 44.

7. "Declaration on Euthanasia," p. 12.

8. Ezekiel J. Emanuel, Linda L. Emanuel, and David Orentlicher, "Advance Directives," *JAMA* 266, 18 (November 13, 1991): letter to the editor, 2563.

Chapter 4: The Sanctity of Life and "Principle of Proportionality"

1. Kevin O'Rourke, "Unfinished Business in the Cruzan Case," *Parameters in Health Care* 16, 1 (St. Louis: St. Louis University Medical Center, 1991), p. 12.

2. *Guidelines*, pp. 6, 9.

3. "Declaration on Euthanasia," p. 10. Direct quotation of Pius XII is from Pius XII, *Address*, February 24, 1957; AAS 49 (1957), p. 147.

4. *Guidelines*, p. 19.

5. Richard A. McCormick, "Theology and Bioethics," *The Hastings Center Report* (March/April 1989): 10.

6. "Declaration on Euthanasia," p. 12.

7. Ibid., pp. 11, 13.

8. "The Covenant of Life and the Caring Community," received by The 195th General Assembly (Louisville: The Office of the General Assembly, 1983), pp. 23-24. Hereafter referred to as "The Covenant of Life."

9. Daniel Callahan, "Medical Futility, Medical Necessity: The Problem-Without-A-Name," *The Hastings Center Report* 21, 4 (July/August 1991): 33.

Chapter 5: Unresolved Ethical Issues

1. William A. Karis, "The Incompetent Developmentally Disabled Person's Right of Self-Determination: Right-to-Die, Sterilization and Institutionalization," *American Journal of Law and Medicine* 15, 2-3, 352.

2. Clarence J. Sundram, "Informed Consent for Major Medical Treatment of Mentally Disabled People: A New Approach," *New England Journal of Medicine* 318, 21 (May 26, 1988): 1368-73.

3. *Conservatorship of Drabick*, at 200 Cal. App. 3d at 205.

4. "Proposed Guidelines of Foregoing Life-Sustaining Treatment" (approved 5/89), developed by the Joint Committee on Bioethics of the San Diego County Medical Society and San Diego County Bar Association, p. 9.

5. "Principles and Guidelines Concerning the Foregoing of Life-Sustaining Treatment for Adult Patients," Joint Committee on Bioethics, Los Angeles County Medical Association, Los Angeles County Bar Association, February 1990, pp. 6-7.

6. *Barber v. Superior Court*, 146 Cal. App. 3d 106 (1983), Drabick, 200 Cal. App. ed at 209.

7. Drs. Steinbrook and Lo, "Artificial Feeding—Solid Ground, Not a Slippery Slope," *The New England Journal of Medicine* 318, 5 (February 4, 1988): 288.

8. Kevin O'Rourke, "The A.M.A. Statement on Tube Feeding: An Ethical Analysis," *America* (November 22, 1986): 322.

9. Robert Barry, "Feeding the Comatose and the Common Good in the Catholic Tradition," *The Thomist* 53, 1 (January 1989): 30.

10. Rev. James J. McCartney, "Catholic Positions on Withholding Sustenance for the Terminally Ill" (Published by The Catholic Health Association of the United States, 1986). Reprinted from *Health Progress*.

Chapter 6: "Advance Directives" for Informed Consent

1. Ernest Becker, *The Denial of Death* (New York: The Free Press, 1973), pp. 22, 26.

2. Allen Benson, "How Will I Die?" *New England Journal of Medicine* 324, 16 (April 18, 1991): 1140.

Chapter 7: How to Decide: Advance Directives

1. "The Medical Directive" (1) Copyright 1990 by Linda L. Emanuel and Ezekiel J. Emanuel. The authors of this form advise that it should be completed pursuant to a discussion between the principal and his or her physician, so that the principal can be adequately informed of any pertinent medical information, and so that the physician can be appraised of the intentions of the principal and the existence of such a document which may be made part of the principal's medical records. (2) This form was originally published as part of an article by Linda L. Emanuel and Ezekiel J. Emanuel, "The Medical Directive: A New Comprehensive Advance Care Document" in *Journal of the American Medical Association* (June 9, 1989): 261:3290. It does not reflect the official policy of the American Medical Association.

Chapter 9: Christian Belief and Treatment Decisions

1. Daniel Callahan, "Religion and the Secularization of Bioethics," *The Hastings Center Report* (July/August 1990): 4.
2. Courtney S. Campbell and Daniel Callahan, eds., "Theology, Religious Traditions, and Bioethics," a special supplement to The Hastings Center Report (July/August 1990): 9.
3. *Webster's New Collegiate Dictionary* (Springfield, Mass.: G. & C. Merriam Company, 1989), p. 227.
4. Marcus J. Borg, *Jesus: A New Vision* (New York: Harper & Row, 1987), p. 65.
5. "The Covenant of Life," pp. 23-24.

Chapter 11: Some Thoughts for Pastoral Care Givers and Religious Professionals

1. Egilde P. Seravalli, "The Dying Patient, the Physician, and the Fear of Death," *The New England Journal of Medicine* 319, 26 (December 29, 1988): 1729.
2. Howard J. Parad and Libbie G. Parad, eds., *Crisis Intervention, Book 2: The Practitioner's Sourcebook for Grief Therapy* (Milwaukee: Family Service America, 1990), pp. 280-87.
3. Barbara Hills LesStrang, *Afterloss: A Recovery Companion for Those Who Are Grieving* (Nashville: Thomas Nelson Publishers, 1992), p. 207.

About the Author

Joseph E. Beltran is an ordained minister in the Presbyterian Church (USA) and works as the Protestant Chaplain at Fairview Developmental Center, a residential center for the developmentally disabled in the state of California. Dr. Beltran is chairperson of Fairview's bioethics committee and serves on the steering committee of the Orange County Bioethics Committee. Dr. Beltran has extensive theoretical and practical experience in the field of bioethics.

Dr. Beltran is a graduate of Whittier College (B.A.), Princeton Theological Seminary (M.Div.) and San Francisco Theological Seminary (D.Min.).